Fine Needle Aspiration Biopsy of the Liver

Fine Needle Aspiration Biopsy of the Liver

A Color Atlas

Martha Bishop Pitman, M.D.

Assistant Pathologist and Director of Fine Needle
Aspiration Biopsy Service, Massachusetts General Hospital
Instructor, Harvard Medical School
Boston, Massachusetts

Wanda Maria Szyfelbein, M.D.

Associate Pathologist, Massachusetts General Hospital
Assistant Professor of Pathology, Harvard Medical School
Boston, Massachusetts

Provided as an educational service by:

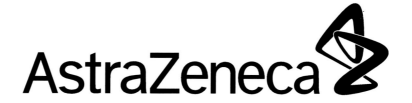

Butterworth–Heinemann
Boston   London   Oxford   Singapore   Sydney   Toronto   Wellington

Library of Congress Cataloging-in-Publication Data

Fine needle aspiration biopsy of the liver : a color atlas / [edited by] Martha Bishop
  Pitman and Wanda Maria Szyfelbein.
    p. cm.
  Includes bibliographical references and index.
  ISBN 0-7506-9463-7
  1. Liver—Needle biopsy—Atlases.   I. Pitman, Martha Bishop.
  II. Szyfelbein, Wanda Maria.
  [DNLM: 1. Biopsy, Needle—methods—atlases. 2. Liver Neoplasms—
    diagnosis—atlases. 3. Liver Diseases—diagnosis—atlases. WI 17
  F495 1994]
  RC847.5.B56F54 1994
  616.3′620758—dc20
  DNLM/DLC
  for Library of Congress   94–15909
                                                                         CIP

British Library Cataloguing-in-Publication Data
A catalogue record for this book is available from the British Library.

Butterworth–Heinemann
313 Washington Street
Newton, MA 02158

10 9 8 7 6 5 4 3 2

Printed in the United States of America

*To the memory of my father, George Benjamin Bishop,
a generous and loving man*

MBP

*To the memory of my beloved parents,
Kazimierz and Janina Kozlicki*

WMS

Contributors

Peter Mueller, M.D.
Division Head, Abdominal Imaging and Interventional Radiology,
Massachusetts General Hospital; Associate Professor of Radiology,
Harvard Medical School, Boston, Massachusetts

Peter Eisenberg, M.D.
Clinical Assistant in Radiology, Massachusetts General Hospital,
Boston, Massachusetts

Giles Boland, M.D.
Clinical Assistant in Radiology, Massachusetts General Hospital,
Boston, Massachusetts

Christine Chmura, CT (ASCP)
Cytology Laboratory, Massachusetts General Hospital,
Boston, Massachusetts

Contents

Preface

This monograph is intended for physicians, fellows, residents, cytotechnologists, and students who are presently involved with or are interested in learning about fine needle aspiration biopsy (FNAB) of the liver. The information in the text is succinct and meant only as a general overview and supplement to the illustrations, the features of which we describe in detail. This monograph is not intended to be an all-encompassing textbook on liver biopsy techniques or liver pathology, but is simply a color atlas of many of the diseases, both benign and malignant, that can affect the liver and that may be encountered on FNAB.

The procedures described for both imaging and processing are those we follow at Massachusetts General Hospital. We attempt to obtain both aspirate smear and cell block material on all specimens if feasible. Rapid interpretations are provided on all biopsies and are made on modified hematoxylin & eosin stained smears, hence, the variety of stains and colors in the illustrations. The cell block preparations, in most cases, complement the smears

nicely; in other cases they may be nondiagnostic of the lesion, or at times, the only diagnostic material available. They are most helpful in making a definitive diagnosis of the non- neoplastic and benign neoplastic lesions. Cell block preparations or core biopsies alone, however, are much less desirable than aspirate smears alone if forced to choose. This is primarily due to the decreased sampling error provided by aspiration biopsy, which can usually be performed multiple times without increased complications, enabling the lesion to be thoroughly sampled.

Fine needle aspiration biopsy of all areas of the body continues to grow in popularity due to its ease, efficiency, and cost-effectiveness. In these changing times of health care reform, we, as physicians, are having to do more with less, and FNAB is one way we can help minimize costs while maintaining excellence in diagnostic care.

MBP and WMS

Acknowledgments

We are grateful to Drs. Peter R. Mueller, Peter J. Eisenberg, and Giles W. Boland for their expertise and contributions of Chapters 1 and 2, and to Christine Chmura for her contribution of Chapter 3.

Special thanks go to Joyce Cheatham for her secretarial assistance and to Steve Conly and Michelle Forrestall for their photographic assistance.

We appreciate the generous contributions of photographs from Drs. Fiona Graeme-Cook, Carolyn Compton, and Robert H. Young of the Massachusetts General Hospital, and from the American Society of Clinical Pathologists.

Last, but not least, we extend our many thanks to our families and our pathology department for their support.

PART

I

Overview of Fine Needle Aspiration Biopsy of the Liver

Introduction

*Peter J. Eisenberg, Giles W. Boland, and
Peter R. Mueller*

Needle biopsy has been used as a method for tissue diagnosis since the early 1900s, well before the development of the sophisticated imaging techniques now routinely used to improve diagnostic accuracy.[1] Martin and Ellis first described the cytologic analysis of samples of solid tumors obtained by percutaneous needle aspiration using an 18-gauge needle in 1934.[2] Initially, the technique was not used in the diagnosis of intra-abdominal disease, and it was not until the 1960s that interest in it was renewed after Lundquist and others demonstrated that cytodiagnosis of material obtained from fine needle aspiration compared favorably with the final histologic diagnoses of specimens obtained at surgery.[3] Fine needle aspiration biopsy (FNAB) first was used only in the diagnosis of malignant disease. Now the technique is routinely used in the diagnosis of benign disease as well. Developments in cross-sectional imaging, advances in cytologic techniques, and new biopsy needles have contributed to a rapid increase in the use of radiologically guided FNAB of the liver.[4] The procedure is widely accepted as safe, efficacious, and accurate.[5] Confident diagnosis can be made in more than 90 percent of cases, including evaluation of lesions as small as 0.5 cm.[6] As the technique has advanced, its limiting factor has become the resolution of available imaging modalities.

INDICATIONS

In the majority of cases, percutaneous FNAB of the liver is performed to confirm the diagnosis of suspected malignancy. It allows the physician to move beyond the limits of differential diagnosis and provides tissue to make a specific diagnosis.[7] Patients with a previous history of malignancy and liver lesions and patients with focal liver abnormalities are prime candidates for percutaneous biopsy. Percutaneous liver biopsy is frequently used for histologic staging to direct further patient management. For example, plans for attempted curative surgery may be changed to a palliative procedure if a biopsy demonstrates previously unsuspected metastatic disease to the liver. Similarly, a diagnosis of a benign focal liver abnormality such as focal nodular hyperplasia or fatty infiltration may eliminate the need for surgical diagnosis.

CONTRAINDICATIONS

Contraindications to FNAB of the liver are few. The first is an uncorrectable bleeding diathesis such as in a patient with thrombocytopenia or markedly abnormal coagulation parameters.[4] Even these conditions may be considered a relative contraindication. Although one might expect greater potential for bleeding complications with large gauge needles, this tendency has not necessarily been proven in clinical practice or in animal studies. Studies using an animal model demonstrated no significant difference in the blood loss experienced using 18-, 20-, or 22-gauge needles between a control group and animals treated with anticoagulants.[7]

The second contraindication to the procedure is the lack of a safe access route to the lesion, as in a biopsy through a vascular structure. This contraindication may also be relative as occasionally the marginal benefit of an FNAB diagnosis of a splenic lesion, for example, may be greater than the potential for bleeding. This potential danger becomes less of a problem as radiologists become more versatile with the multiplanar capabilities of computed tomography and ultrasound-guided procedures.

A third contraindication is an uncooperative patient. Most large and superficial lesions may be biopsied with minimal patient cooperation. However, small inaccessible lesions may require the patient to assume awkward positions and maintain strict breath control to assure consistent needle passage along the planned trajectory. While the risk of bleeding is slight in most patients, uncontrolled motion during the procedure may lead to needle transgression across major vascular structures, as well as out of the optimal biopsy plane.[8]

Fine needle aspiration biopsy has proven safe even in such diverse lesions as hemangioma and *Echinococcus granulosa*.[9] As with all FNAB, the potential risk must be measured against the benefit.

ADVANTAGES

There are many advantages to FNAB of the liver. As noted by Bret, et al.,[10] the results of FNAB can contribute to a decrease in the total number of tests, especially invasive ones, and a decrease in the length of hospital stay of patients, which may result in significant cost savings. In their evaluation of 112 abdominal lesions, including 69 of the liver, it was concluded that 34 laparoscopies, 11 exploratory laparotomies, and 14 angiograms were avoided for the group as a whole due to the FNAB.[10]

Another advantage of FNAB with rapid cytologic analysis is that the adequacy of the biopsy specimen can be determined during the procedure—before the patient is discharged—so that additional passes or a different type of needle or technique can be used if the initial biopsy is nondiagnostic.[11]

A further advantage is that if a differential diagnosis is entertained at the time of initial biopsy, additional material may be obtained and fixed appropriately for the specific studies or stains that the cytopathologist may deem necessary.[12]

PREBIOPSY ASSESSMENT

As noted by Murphy et al.,[13] the purpose of preprocedure testing is to discover abnormalities that subject patients to an increased risk of complications so that one may reduce the risk to an acceptable level. The use of preprocedure hemostatic evaluation as a routine is controversial. A reasonable approach to preprocedure screening has been proposed by Silverman, et al.[14] Their review states that the primary means for identifying a patient with higher potential for bleeding complications is the patient's clinical history. By their methodology, if a patient has a normal screening history the only routine testing of hemostatic function should include a partial thromboplastin time and platelet count. These examina-

tions should detect an unsuspected anticoagulant disorder—for example, thrombocytopenia or occult disseminated intravascular coagulation. Additional studies of hemostasis are dictated by the abnormalities discovered during a thorough screening history or in patients with a known or suspected hemostatic defect.[14]

The issue of performing FNAB in patients who have a history of using aspirin and other nonsteroidal anti-inflammatory drugs that have antiplatelet actions remains controversial. The most conservative approach would be to delay the procedure for 3 to 10 days after the last dose of aspirin. However, if the biopsy cannot be delayed the radiologist and referring clinicians must accept the hemostatic defect and, relying on the absence of any evidence of associated defects, accept that the statistical likelihood that a significant hemorrhagic complication will result from the aspirin use is probably very low.[14]

An extremely important part of the prebiopsy preparation includes considering the psychological needs of the patient both during and after the procedure. Patients scheduled for interventional procedures arrive with a high level of anxiety about the pain they fear may result from the procedure as well as the possibility of abnormal results. This anxiety may adversely affect their ability to cooperate with difficult instructions and increases the risk of complications. Spending a brief period of time with the patient before the procedure gives the radiologist an opportunity to explain the necessity as well as the actual mechanics and possible complications of the procedure.

Additional factors to be addressed in the prebiopsy assessment are how the size of the patient relates to patient positioning, the choice of the most appropriate imaging modality to be used for the procedure, the size and location of the lesion(s) of interest, tumor vascularity, and any special equipment that may be needed based on body habitus or other patient specific requirements.[6,8] Appropriate prebiopsy assessment including review of the imaging studies prior to the biopsy allows for the most efficient use of valuable hospital and physician resources.

BIOPSY COMPLICATIONS

Although FNAB of the liver is considered to be safe, it is not entirely free of complications. Several long-term follow-up studies have demonstrated a very low rate of serious complications.[9] Literature reviews have noted mortality rates following fine needle biopsy of the abdomen from 0.006 to 0.1 percent. Bleeding after biopsy of liver lesions may be due to the vascularity of the lesion, the location of the lesion, or the needle size used. For example, bleeding after biopsy of hemangioma has been reported when the hemangioma was peripheral (pericapsular) in location. Several authors have suggested attempting to biopsy vascular lesions through normal liver tissue to avoid this serious complication.[9]

Review of the literature reveals only three reported cases of needle tract seeding following liver biopsy using noncutting needles.[9] The estimated rate of needle tract seeding following FNAB of all abdominal organs ranges from 0.003 to 0.009 percent.[9] The actual rate of needle tract seeding may be higher, as there is a considerable time interval between biopsy and the subsequent development of metastatic lesions. Various factors such as the number of cells dislodged, cellular adhesiveness, enzymatic release, the amount of stroma present, and individual patient immunologic factors may all relate to needle tract seeding.[15]

An additional rare, albeit reported, complication following FNAB of the liver is fatal carcinoid crisis after biopsy of a hepatic metastasis.[12] Carcinoid tumors and pheochromocytomas represent hormonally active lesions with unstable release patterns. The mechanism of hormonal release is not completely understood and may be associated with increased intratumoral pressure related to hemorrhage and massive hormonal release into the systemic circulation.[16]

As a result of these few but significant potential complications, FNAB should be performed only when indicated and after appropriate precautions have been taken. Rapid analysis of cytological material should be available, and the number of needle "passes" should be kept to the minimum consistent with the needs to obtain diagnostic material.

REFERENCES

1. Guthrie CG. Gland puncture as a diagnostic measure. Bull Johns Hopkins Hosp 1921;32:266.

2. Martin HE, Ellis EB. Aspiration Biopsy. Surg Gynecol Obstet 1934;59:578–582.

3. Lundquist A: Fine-needle aspiration biopsy of the liver. Acta Med Scand[Suppl] 1971;520:1–28.

4. Hopper KD, Abendroth CS, Sturtz KW, Matthews YL, Shirk SJ. Fine-needle aspiration biopsy for cytopathologic analysis: utility of syringe handles, auto-mated guns, and the nonsuction method. Radiology 1992;185:819–824.

5. Welch TJ, Sheedy PF, Johnson CD, Johnson CM, Stephens DH. CT-guided biopsy: prospective analysis of 1,000 procedures. Radiology 1989;171:493–496.

6. Charboneau JW, Reading CC, Welch TJ. CT and sonographically guided needle biopsy: current techniques and new interventions. AJR Am J Roentgenol 1990;154:1–10.

7. Gazelle GS, Haaga JR, Rowland DY. Effect of needle gauge, level of anticoagulation, and target organ on bleeding associated with aspiration biopsy (work in progress). Radiology 1992;183:509–513.

8. Ferrucci JT, et al. Interventional radiology of the abdomen. 2nd ed. Baltimore: Williams & Wilkins, 1985;36–46.

9. Smith EH. Complications of percutaneous abdominal fine-needle biopsy. Radiology 1991;178:253–258.

10. Bret PM, Fond A, Casola G, Bretagnolle M, Germain-Lacour MJ, Bret P, Labadie, M, Buffard P. Abdominal lesions: a prospective study of clinical efficacy of percutaneous fine-needle biopsy. Radiology 1986;159:345–346.

11. Lees WR, Hall-Craggs MA, Manhire A. Five years' experience of fine needle aspiration biopsy: 454 consecutive cases. Clin Radiol 1985;36:517–520.

12. Fagelman D, Chess Q. Nonaspiration fine-needle cytology of the liver: a new technique for obtaining diagnostic samples. AJR Am J Roentgenol 1990; 155: 1217–1219.

13. Murphy TP, Dorfman GS, Becker J. Use of preprocedural tests by interventional radiologists. Radiology 1993;186:213–220.

14. Silverman SG, Mueller PR, Pfister RC. Hemostatic evaluation before abdominal interventions: an overview and proposal. AJR Am J Roentgenol 1990;154: 233– 238.

15. Weiss H. Metostasebildung durch feinnadelpunktion? Ultra schall Med 1988;10:147–151.

16. Bissonnette RT, Gibney RG, Berry BR, Buckley AR. Fatal carcinoid crisis after percutaneous fine-needle biopsy of hepatic metastasis: case report and literature review. Radiology 1990;174:751–752.

CHAPTER

2

Biopsy Techniques

Giles W. Boland, Peter J. Eisenberg, and
Peter R. Mueller

IMAGE GUIDANCE SYSTEMS

Two major factors influence the choice of the radiologic guidance systems used to perform fine needle aspiration biopsy (FNAB): (1) the size and location of the lesion in the liver and (2) the personal preference and previous experience of the radiologist performing the procedure. Ideally the location and size of the lesion should determine which modality is used, but in practice, personal preference may decide which modality is used, as the accuracy for needle biopsy improves with experience. In general, ultrasound is used as the initial guidance system, particularly for diffuse multiple lesions and for large superficial lesions. Computed tomography (CT) is used if the lesion is small or not easily visualized by ultrasound.

Ultrasound

The major advantage of sonographic biopsy guidance is its ability to visualize the needle in multiple planes and provide continuous real-time needle localization within the liver. With experience the procedure is quick and, if necessary, can be performed at the bedside. Other advantages include the lack of ionizing radiation and relative low cost compared to CT. Any structures that attenuate the ultrasound beam such as fat and air will reduce visualization of the needle. For this reason, sonographically guided liver biopsies may be difficult to perform in obese patients and in patients with fatty replacement of the liver. Intervening lung or bowel gas may make it impossible to see the biopsy needle. Similarly, the needle may be difficult to visualize in deeply seated lesions due to sound attenuation through the liver. Perhaps the most important limiting factor to sonographic-guided biopsy is operator skill. It is technically more difficult to perform than CT-guided biopsy, and considerable experience with real-time scanning is necessary before the physician becomes successful.

Advances in ultrasound transducer technology in recent years has made biopsy technically easier. Electronic phased-array transducers provide better needle visualization than mechanical scanners. A linear-array transducer has a wider field of view for the initial portion of the needle than does the narrow near field of a sector scanner, but sector scanners are required if intervening ribs provide a narrow acoustic window.

Modifications have been made to the transducer body to facilitate needle localization within the liver.[1] These include a detachable guide that directs the needle to specific depths within the liver. Some transducers have built-in needle slots within which biopsy needles of various gauges are positioned and that direct the needle into a predetermined angle within the plane of view of the transducer. Most radiologists, however, prefer the "free-hand" technique, which requires greater operator skill but is ideally suited to real-time scanning and allows greatest flexibility to the radiologist.[2] With the freehand technique, the ultrasound transducer is held in one hand and the biopsy needle is directed to the lesion with the other hand. As with all sonographically guided needle techniques, the needle must be positioned in the long axis of the ultrasound beam. Failure to clearly visualize the needle usually indicates that the needle has been either initially aligned off-center relative to the central beam of

FIGURE 2–1 Ultrasound biopsy demonstrating 18-gauge needle (*arrow*) at the periphery of the lesion.

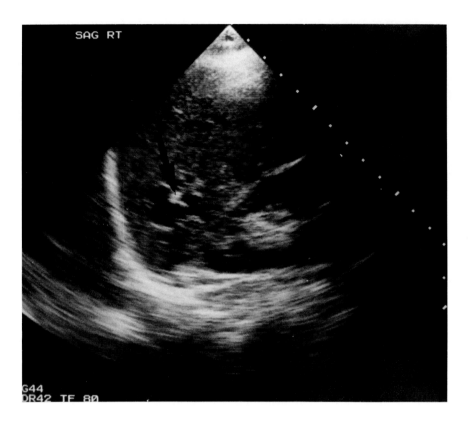

the transducer or angled across the main axis of the beam and out of the field of view of the transducer. Fine jiggling in and out movements of the needle aid needle localization. Minor freehand adjustments to the needle allow accurate needle placement within the lesion and compensate for patient breathing and minor needle mis-alignments[1](Figure 2–1).

Due to the changing position of the liver during respiration, small lesions are more suited to ultrasound guidance so that continuous monitoring of the needle is possible. Lesions located in the dome of the liver can be biopsied by ultrasound guidance as a steep angle of approach is required to avoid the lung. Caudal lesions can be approached subcostally or intercostally.

Computed Tomography

CT-guided biopsy is technically easier to perform than that using ultrasound guidance but is usually a more lengthy procedure. It is a well-established technique and is the imaging modality of choice in some institutions. Unlike ultrasound, the presence of intestinal gas or over-lying bone rarely impedes CT localization of hepatic lesions. The main advantage of CT is the ability to clearly visualize the needle within the lesion, which at times can be difficult with ultrasound guidance.

After initial CT scanning has localized a hepatic lesion, several CT slices are performed with a lead grid on the skin overlying the approximate intended needle

trajectory to the lesion. The precise site of entry through the skin is then marked with a pen, the grid is removed, and the needle is inserted to a predetermined depth and location avoiding vital organs such as lung and colon. Usually the needle should be advanced in a plane per-fectly parallel to and within the center of the x-ray beam. In this way the needle tip is clearly identified as an abrupt end to the needle and is associated with a black metallic artifact beyond the needle tip in the soft tissues (Figure 2–2). Any angulation out of the plane of the x-ray beam will create difficulties in identifying the needle tip, and multiple scans and needle repositions are required to determine the correct angle and depth of insertion. An angled needle shaft is recognized by a tapered rather than abrupt appearance and does not have an associated artifact (Figure 2–3). Occasionally an oblique path to the lesion is specifically chosen to avoid the lung, although transpleural biopsies with small needles are associated with few complications. Unlike ultrasound, real-time monitoring of the needle is not possible with CT, and several passes with repeat scanning may be required before the needle path is accurately directed to the lesion.

NEEDLE SELECTION

A large variety of needle calibers, lengths, and tip designs are available for effectively performing biopsies to retrieve cytologic material. Needles can be divided into smaller (20–22) or larger (18) gauges.[3] Needles

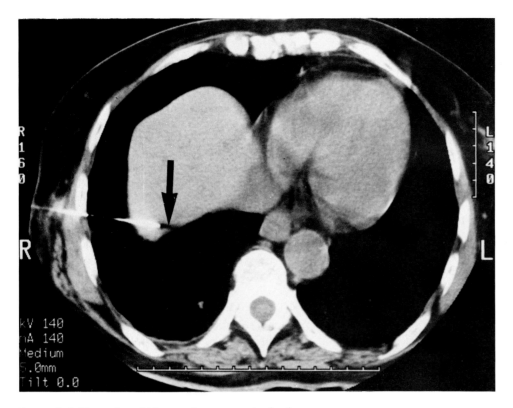

FIGURE 2–2 Transpleural biopsy of metastases in the dome of the liver. The needle tip is identified by an abrupt end to the needle with associated black metallic artifact beyond the needle tip (*arrow*).

FIGURE 2–3 The same patient as in Figure 2–2 before repositioning the needle. The needle tip is identified by a tapered end without a black metallic artifact, indicating the needle is not perpendicular to the x-ray beam.

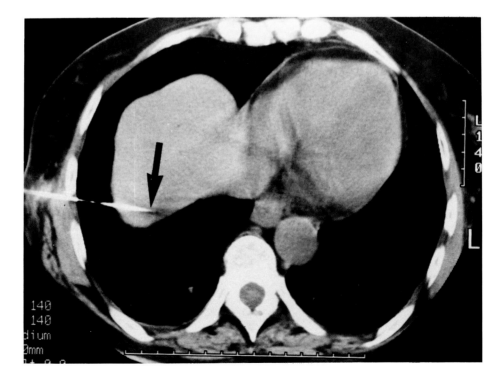

larger than 18 gauge are generally not used for aspiration cytology biopsy. Smaller-gauge needles are traditionally considered safer than larger needles, although no controlled trial has evaluated the relative complication rate in humans. However, there is little risk in puncturing vascular and intestinal structures with small-gauge needles, and multiple passes can therefore be made. These needles can usually retrieve an adequate tissue sample for cytologic analysis. A fragment or tissue core can often be retrieved for histology, but smaller needles are less consistent in obtaining adequate tissue for histology than larger needles.

Small-gauge Needles

Small-gauge needles are associated with little risk and therefore allow multiple punctures. These needles are particularly useful when the biopsy route traverses the pleura, vascular structures, and bowel. They offer a greater safety margin in the presence of a bleeding diathesis. Although small-gauge needles can often confirm tumor recurrence or metastases of known previous malignancy, larger tissue cores are sometimes required for reliable diagnosis of certain tumors if the type of malignancy is unknown. Thinner 22-gauge needles may also meet substantial resistance and therefore bend when biopsying a firm, solid tumor or normal calcified structures. Twenty-gauge needles offer similar safety features but obtain slightly larger tissue fragments and allow greater control and penetration from the stiffer shaft. We therefore perform our initial localization with a 22-gauge reference needle placement and use 20-gauge needles for subsequent biopsies.

Larger-gauge Needles

If initial use of a 20-gauge needle does not provide enough cytologic material, a subsequent biopsy with an 18-gauge needle is made using a 22-gauge reference needle. The risk of hemorrhage is slightly higher than with thin-gauge needles and therefore biopsy should be limited to fewer passes. Larger-gauge needles significantly improve the rate of recovering cytologic and histologic material compared to thinner gauge needles, and therefore only one or two passes generally are required. Some institutions perform the majority of both CT- and sonogram-guided biopsies with 18-gauge needles, a practice that combines a high cytologic and histologic recovery rate with relatively low complication rates.

Needle Design

Modifications have been made to the conventional 22-gauge Chiba needle in an attempt to cut better tissue cores. The tip of the needle, the bevel angle, and the edge

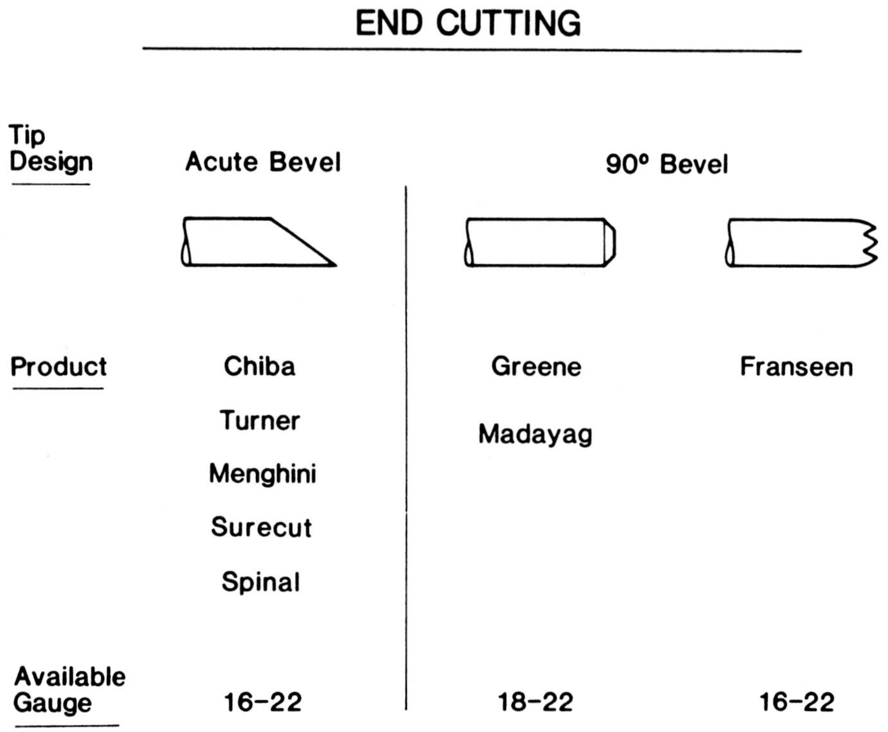

FIGURE 2–4 Schematic representation of needle tip designs demonstrating variation in bevel and cutting edge. (Reprinted in part from JT Ferrucci, J Wittenberg, P Mueller, J Simeone, eds. Interventional radiology of the abdomen. Baltimore: William & Wilkins 1985;47. With permission.)

END CUTTING

Tip Design	Acute Bevel	90° Bevel	
Product	Chiba Turner Menghini Surecut Spinal	Greene Madayag	Franseen
Available Gauge	16–22	18–22	16–22

of the bevel can be modified to various degrees (Figure 2–4).

Needles are available in several different lengths, the choice of which should depend on the depth of the lesion to be biopsied. When biopsying a superficial lesion, a shorter needle avoids needle tilt or movement, which occurs when too much shaft of the needle remains outside the body. In addition, the diameter of the CT gantry orifice may not accommodate a long needle, particularly if the patient is obese. Longer needles will be required for deeper biopsies.

PERFORMING THE BIOPSY

Needle Insertion

Both operator and patient should be comfortable before the biopsy. Most biopsies can be done with the patient in the supine position, but occasionally an oblique or lateral decubitus position is necessary to bring the lesion into a more suitable position for biopsy. The site of the needle entry is usually the shortest distance from the skin to the lesion, although a longer path may be required to avoid lung or intervening bowel and vascular structures.

Adequate patient sedation is essential to avoid sudden undue patient movement, which significantly increases the technical difficulty in performing the biopsy. The skin is first cleansed with povidone-iodine or alcohol. If ultrasound biopsy is being performed, the transducer can be covered with a sterile sheath, but this can degrade the image, and it is less cumbersome to simply sterilize the transducer probe directly. Ultrasound biopsies can be performed with gentle respiration as the needle can be visualized real-time relative to the lesion. The skin and subcutaneous tissues are anesthetized to and including the liver capsule.

Biopsies can be performed with either a single- or two-needle technique. The two-needle technique involves an initial needle placement that either acts as a reference to subsequent needle placements (tandem technique)[4] or as a guide in which a biopsy can be performed by placement of one needle through another (coaxial technique).[4] The depth of the proximal margin of the lesion from the skin surface is measured and the needle is advanced to the precise depth. Considerable patience is required to angle the needle correctly so that the needle can be adequately monitored (either by CT or ultrasound) as it is advanced. With the single-needle technique, multiple passes are made into the mass. Most biopsies in our institution are performed with the two-needle tandem technique. Meticulous care is required to position the reference needle at the proximal margin of the mass as subsequent tandem needles of larger gauge (18–20) are placed immediately beside this needle; their position should not need to be confirmed by further imaging. Multiple passes with the reference needle may be required before its position can be considered adequate. Once the reference needle tip is satisfactorily placed within the mass, the precise distance from the skin to the proximal tumor margin is measured and the tandem needle is inserted the identical depth as the reference needle.

The coaxial technique involves initial insertion of an 18- or 19-gauge needle to the proximal margin of the tumor. The stylet is removed and a longer, thinner-gauge needle is advanced through and beyond the larger needle. Usually several aspirations are performed with the thinner-gauge needle and a final aspiration is taken with the larger needle. The coaxial technique is suited to biopsy of lesions in deep or difficult locations, as precise needle placement is only required once, reducing the risk of hemorrhage.

Tissue Sampling

The exact mechanism for obtaining tissue begins by attaching a 12-cc syringe to the hub of the needle. To provide a core biopsy a rotatory or "drilling motion" is applied to the barrel of the syringe by the fingers of one hand while suction and insertion are controlled with the other hand.[4] A Luer-Lok® device is preferable for maximum needle responsiveness during rotation and aspiration, which is created with suction by withdrawal of the plunger. The syringe is rotated continuously in a cork-boring manner as the needle is advanced through the lesion. As the needle is inserted, blood may be aspirated or alternatively no visible aspirate is seen. The tissue sample usually lodges within the needle shaft itself and is only appreciated after the syringe is removed and its contents expelled onto the slide. The needle is withdrawn after releasing suction to avoid aspirating normal intervening tissue and air. The syringe is then removed from the needle and a few cc's of air are drawn into the syringe. It is reconnected to the needle, and the tissue sample is gently expelled onto a slide. Any particulate fragments are placed in saline for histologic analysis.

False-negative aspiration biopsies can be minimized by performing multiple biopsies using either the single- or double-needle technique, which reduces needle sampling error of necrotic, hemorrhagic, or inflammatory material within the lesion. However, meticulous attention to patient positioning, choice of imaging modality, needle selection, and biopsy technique are essential to maximize the recovery of suitable tissue for subsequent cytologic analysis.

REFERENCES

1. Charboneau JW, Reading CC, Welch TJ. CT and sonographically guided needle biopsy: current techniques and new innovations. AJR Am J Roentgenol 1990; 154:1–10.

2. Reading CC, Charboneau JW, James EM, Hurt MR. Sonographically guided percutaneous biopsy of small (3 cm or less) masses. AJR Am J Roentgenol 1988; 151:189–192.

3. Lieberman RP, Hafez GR, Crummy AB. Histology from aspiration biopsy: Turner needle experience. AJR Am J Roentgenol 1982;138:561–564.

4. Wittenberg J, Mueller PR, Ferrucci JT, et al. Percutaneous core biopsy of abdominal tumors using 22 gauge needles: further observations. AJR Am J Roentgenol 1982;139:75–80.

3

Specimen Preparatory Techniques

Christine Chmura

At Massachusetts General Hospital rapid interpretation of all radiologically guided biopsies is performed. The role of the cytotechnologist is exciting and challenging as he or she is the first to arrive on the scene. The cytotechnologist must rapidly prepare the slides and evaluate specimen adequacy. The cytopathologist then issues a statement of adequacy, a preliminary diagnosis, and if necessary, requests tissue for special studies such as for a lymphoma work-up.

CLINICAL INFORMATION

In our laboratory, great emphasis is placed on obtaining the patient's clinical diagnosis and history. Before evaluating the aspiration, we obtain past diagnoses via previous cytology and pathology reports, treatment history, and any available relevant glass slides for comparison. Important current clinical information includes the size of the lesion, whether it is single or one of multiple nodules, whether the clinical suspicion is of a primary lesion or a metastasis, radiologic findings, and relevant serologic studies (e.g., alphafetoprotein levels). The gathering of this history is vital for an accurate rapid interpretation.

PREPARATION OF RAPID SMEARS

The cytotechnologist travels to the designated area in radiology when alerted by the radiology department. A mobile aspiration staining kit is carried to the reading room, where a temporary lab is set up. Microscopes are conveniently stored there for our purposes. The contents of the aspiration biopsy kit include water baths, stains, xylene, mounting media, coverslips, paper clips (which keep slides separate in the jar of alcohol fixative), gauze pads (to drain excess xylene and mounting media), and dotting pens.

After each aspiration biopsy, the radiologist expresses a small amount of the specimen (about 2 drops) on a frosted glass slide. The specimen is smeared using the pull-apart method,[1] as it is the method our cytotechnologists are most familiar and comfortable with, but any smear technique that provides well-preserved, noncrushed material can be used. A clean frosted slide is placed over the one containing the specimen and the material is gently pressed together so as not to crush the sample or strip nuclei of their cytoplasm. The cellular material is pulled away from the labeled end. The two slides are pulled apart and immediately immersed in a fixative of 5 percent glacial acetic acid and 95 percent ethyl alcohol, which achieves rapid fixation and lysis of excess blood. Paper clips are used to keep the slides separated in the jar of fixative. The slides are fixed for a minimum of 30 seconds, and one slide from one or more pairs is chosen to be stained on the basis of cellular material and appearance using the rapid hematoxylin and eosin (H & E) staining technique (Table 3–1).

RAPID INTERPRETATION

The cytotechnologist screens the slide(s) for adequacy, appropriateness of anatomic site, and presence of malignancy. If the slide(s) have only benign hepatocytes, the radiologist may choose to reaspirate. Once the slides

TABLE 3–1   Rapid Hematoxylin and Eosin Stain

Procedure	Duration
1. Fix in solution of 5% glacial acetic acid in 95% ethyl alcohol	30 sec.
2. Wash in distilled water	2 dips
3. Rinse in acid water[a]	2 dips
4. Stain in hematoxylin[b]	30 sec.
5. Rinse in distilled water	3 dips
6. Differentiate in acid water	2 dips
7. Blue immediately in tap waters	4–5 dips
8. Wash in distilled water	10 dips
9. Counterstain in eosin[c]	3–5 dips
10. Dehydrate in 95% ethyl alcohol	5 dips
11. Dehydrate in 99% isopropyl alcohol	5 dips
12. Clear in xylene	5–10 dips
13. Coverslip	

[a]Acid water solution: 2 ml glacial acetic acid in 250 ml distilled water.

[b]Hematoxylin: Gill 3 (triple strength) hematoxylin (Lerner Laboratories, Fisher Scientific, Orangeburge, NY). Be sure to add 2–3 ml glacial acetic acid to each 250 ml of fresh dye solution.

[c]Eosin: Eosin Y, 1% alcohol solution (Harelco Brand, EM Diagnostic Systems, Gibbstown, NJ). Dilute with equal volume of 95% ethyl alcohol. Add 2 ml glacial acetic acid to each 250 ml of staining solution.

PREPARATION OF SLIDES FOR FINAL INTERPRETATION

The remainder of the slides not stained with the rapid H & E are labeled with the patient's name and placed in 95 percent ethyl alcohol until they are ready to be stained by the Papanicolaou (Pap) method (Table 3–2). We do not routinely prepare air-dried smears because we think the vast majority of liver lesions are epithelial and require nuclear detail for optimal evaluation. Air-dried smears are prepared only if requested at the time of rapid interpretation. Needle rinsings suspended in saline are collected and processed by using either Cytospin (Shandon Lipshaw, Pittsburgh, PA) or a Thin Prep Processor (Cytyc Corp., Marlborough, MA). For Cytospins, the sample is transferred to centrifuge tubes and centrifuged at 1,500 rpm for 10 minutes. The supernatant is poured off and the cell pellet is resuspended by vortex in 5 ml of Hank's balanced salt solution. Cytospin

are considered potentially diagnostic of a lesion (benign or malignant), the cytotechnologist calls for the cytopathologist, who determines adequacy and renders a rapid interpretation.

TABLE 3–2   Routine Papanicolaou Stain

Station Number	Solution	Time (min)
1.	Running water	1.0
2.	Hematoxylin[a]	2.0
3.	Running water	1.0
4.	Running water	1.0
5.	96% ethanol	2.0
6.	Orange G[b]	1.0
7.	95% ethanol	2.0
8.	Eosin[c]	6.0
9.	95% ethanol	4.0
10.	95% ethanol	3.0
11.	95% ETOH[d]	2.0
12.	99% isopropanol	3.0
13.	Xylene	2.0
14.	Xylene	2.0

[a]Gill hematoxylin stain

Distilled water	710 ml
Ethyl glycol	250 ml
Hematoxylin (C.I. #75290)	2.0 gm
Sodium iodate (NaIO$_3$)	0.2 gm*
Aluminum sulfate (Al$_2$ (SO4)$_3$ H$_2$O)	17.0 gm
Glacial acetic acid	40.0 ml

*Accurate weight of sodium iodate is *critical*!

Mix all ingredients on magnetic sitrrer for 1 hour. All ingredients must be dissolved. Stain may be used immediately.

[b]Orange G stain: Gill formula

1. Stock solution (0.2 M)
   Dissolve 9.05 gm actual dye in 100 ml distilled water. To find actual dye weight:
   wt (gm) = 9.05 gm
          (% dye content of stain)
2. Orange G working solution

0.2 M stock Orange G	10 ml
Phosphotungstic acid	1 gm
95% ethyl alcohol	985 ml
Glacial acetic acid	5 ml

Stain may be used immediately.

[c]Eosinpolychrome: Gill formula

1. Stock solutions
   Dissolve in 100 ml distilled water (70–80°C)

0.4 M light green SF yellowish (CI #42095)	3.17 gm actual dye
0.30 M eosin Y (CI #45380)	20.8 gm actual dye
0.04 M fast green FCF (CI #42053)	3.24 gm actual dye

2. Working solution for slides

0.04 M light green SF yellowish	10 ml
0.30 M eosin Y	20 ml
Phosphotungstic acid	2.0 gm
95% ethyl alcohol	700 ml
Absolute methyl alcohol	250 ml
Glacial acetic acid	20 ml

[d]Change 95% ethanol of Station 11 between staining runs.

chambers are assembled and five to seven drops of the resuspended sample are placed within the chamber, spun for 1 minute at 1,250 rpm, and fixed in 95 percent ethanol. For Thin Prep slides, the sample is transferred to a centrifuge tube and 30 ml of Cytolyt solution are added. The sample is centrifuged at 600 × g for 10 minutes. The supernatant is poured off, and the pellet is resuspended by vortex. If there is no visible pellet, an aliquot of PreservCyt solution should be poured from the vial into the tube, vortex to mix, and the sample poured back into the vial. Two drops of the sample are pipetted into a 20-ml PreservCyt solution vial. The specimen is incubated for 5 minutes. The slide is then made with the Thin Prep Processor. The specimen is fixed in 95 percent ethyl alcohol until it is ready to be stained by the Pap method.

Tissue core fragments that have been obtained are removed and placed into a centrifuge tube. Three to four drops of plasma are added and the specimen is vortexed to resuspend. Three to four drops of thrombin are added. The firm pellet is covered with 10 percent for- malin for fixation and subsequent histologic processing. The needle rinsing fluid can be used for additional Cytospin or Thin Prep slides if an adequate core is available for cell block. These extra slides may be used for special studies if either a cell button is inadequate for cell block or core samples prove inadequate for diagnosis or special studies.

If a cell block is desired from the fluid sample (no visible tissue fragments), the sample is transferred to a centrifuge tube and centrifuged at 1,500 rpm for 10 min- utes. The supernatant is decanted, and three to four drops of plasma are added. The specimen is resuspended by vortex prior to adding three to four drops of thrombin. The firm pellet is covered with 10 percent formalin for fix- ation and subsequent histologic processing.

LYMPHOMA WORK-UP

If lymphoma is suspected, core biopsy specimens are obtained if possible. Tissue cores are preserved in saline and taken to the frozen section lab, where the specimen is either entirely frozen or divided between frozen tissue, B-5 fixed tissue, and formalin. If only a small amount of tissue is available, it is all frozen. An initial frozen section is cut to determine adequacy for immunoperoxidase studies, and then several frozen sec- tions are cut and placed on albumin-covered nonfrosted glass slides and sent to the immunoperoxidase lab for a panel of antibodies requested by the cytopathologist. From the needle rinsing fluid the cytology lab prepares Cytospin slides: one is air dried and stained by the May-Grünwald-Giemsa method (Harleco Brand EM Diag- nostics, Gibbstown, NJ) (Table 3–3), and four to six Cy- tospin slides are processed, dipped in acetone, air dried, and frozen for immunoperoxidase studies if needed. If

TABLE 3–3   May-Grünwald-Giemsa Stain* on plain (nonfrosted) slides only

Procedure	Duration (min)
1. Fixation in 95% ethyl alcohol	1
2. Stain in May-Grünwald solution	10
3. Rinse in running tap water	1
4. Stain in Giemsa* stain	15
5. Rinse in running tap water	1
6. Air dry and coverslip	

*Azure B type to be used (Harleco, Em Diagnostic Systems, Gibbstown, NJ)

the core tissue is adequate, duplicate immunoperoxidase studies are not performed on the Cytospin slides. If the core tissue is not representative of the suspicious lym- phoid lesion but the air-dried Cytospin preparation is, then the frozen Cytospin preparations are stained to determine monoclonality with a small panel of antibod- ies, usually CD3 (leu4; T cell marker), CD22 (Leu14; B cell marker), kappa, and lambda (Table 3–4). If the Cytospin preparations are inadequate, then previously stained smears can be destained to at least confirm that the atypical population of cells is lymphoid. It is imprac- tical to try to determine monoclonality on destained smear preparations.

OTHER SPECIAL STUDIES

Estrogen-Progesterone Receptors

If the lesion is clinically or morphologically sus- picious for metastatic breast cancer, direct smears can be processed for markers of the estrogen-progesterone receptors (Abbott ER-ICA Monoclonal, Abbott Labora- tories, Abbott Park, IL) or gross cystic fluid protein-15 (Signet Laboratories, Dedham, MA).

Electron Microscopy

If the tumor is a poorly differentiated carcinoma, a sarcoma, or other undifferentiated tumor, either a core biopsy or an aspirate specimen can be fixed in glutaral- dehyde for electron microscopy. This procedure is particu- larly helpful for patients who have no known primary malignancy.

DESTAINING

Slides stained by the Pap method or rapid H & E must be destained for some special stains and immuno- cytochemistry (see Table 3–4). Our destaining method is as follows

TABLE 3–4   Special Studies

Stain	Fixative	Slide Type	Use of Destained Pap Smear
Pap	95% ethanol Acid alcohol	Plain or frosted	—
Fontana Masson	95% ethanol Acid alcohol Formalin	Plain or frosted	Yes
Mucicarmine	95% ethanol Acid alcohol Formalin	Plain or frosted	Yes
Periodic Acid-Schiff	95% ethanol Acid alcohol Formalin	Plain or frosted	Yes
Grocott Methanamine Silver	95% ethanol Acid alcohol Formalin	Plain or frosted	Yes
Chromogranin	95% ethanol Acid alcohol Formalin	Plain or frosted	Yes
May-Grünwald-Giemsa	Air dry	Plain	No
Lymphoid series immunocytochemistry (kappa, lambda CD3, IgG, IgM, CD22)	Air dry	Plain	No
Epithelial series immunocytochemistry			Yes
S-100 Keratin (Cam 5.2 and AE1,3) CEA Alpha-fetoprotein Alpha1-antitrypsin Others	Acid, alcohol, or formalin	Plain or frosted Frosted	

1. The coverslip is removed by placing the slide in xylene until it falls off.
2. Two changes of xylene for 3 minutes each.
3. 99 percent isopropyl alcohol for 3 minutes.
4. 95 percent ethyl alcohol and concentrated hydrochloric acid (1 ml hydrochloric acid to 100 ml ethyl alcohol) for 10 to 15 minutes with occasional dipping (check for decolorization and repeat if necessary).
5. Place in distilled water until it is restained with desired special stain.

REFERENCES

1. Takahashi M. Color atlas of cancer cytology. 2nd ed. Tokyo: Igako-Shoin, 1981;74.

Cytomorphology of the Benign Aspirate

CHAPTER

4

Normal Liver

Martha Bishop Pitman and
Wanda Maria Szyfelbein

The functional unit of the liver is referred to as an acinus, a pie-shaped segment of contiguous lobules fed by branches of the portal vein and hepatic artery stemming from the portal tract.[1] The hexagon-shaped lobules (Figure 4–1) are composed of thin trabeculae (one to two cells thick) separated by sinusoids lined by a discontinuous layer of endothelial cells and kupffer cells (Figure 4–2). The lobule has a central vein and is anchored by portal tracts containing a branch of the portal vein, hepatic artery, and one or two interlobular bile ducts. Fibroblasts and occasional lymphocytes surround these structures in the portal tracts (Figure 4–3).

HEPATOCYTES

The components of a normal liver aspirate, then, are primarily hepatocytes and bile duct epithelial cells, with occasional kupffer cells, sinusoidal endothelial cells, mononuclear cells, and fibroblasts. Normal hepatocytes occur as monolayered sheets, small groups, thin (one to two cells) trabeculae, and single cells. They are polygonal

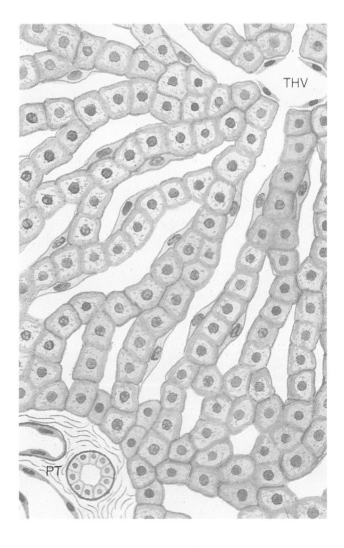

FIGURE 4–1 Schematic diagram of the normal liver lobule showing thin (one to two cells thick) trabeculae separated by sinusoids that drain into a terminal hepatic venule (THV) or central vein and are anchored by portal tracts (PT) containing branches of the hepatic artery, portal vein, and interlobular bile duct. (Reproduced with permission by Dimitri Karetnikov, E Rubin, J Farber, eds. Pathology. Philadelphia: J.B. Lippincott, 1988; p. 725.

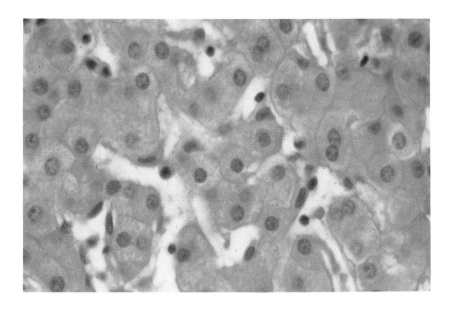

FIGURE 4–2 Normal liver parenchyma on histologic section. Thin (one to two cells) trabeculae are separated by sinusoids lined by discontinuous endothelium and scattered kupffer cells. Hepatocytes contain one or two small- to medium-sized, round, centrally placed nuclei with small but visible nucleoli and abundant eosinophilic, granular cytoplasm. (Hematoxylin & eosin, ×160.)

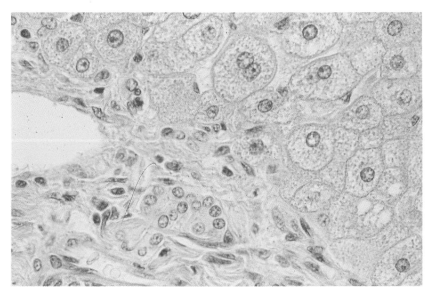

FIGURE 4–3 Normal liver histology of the portal tract with vein, artery, and bile ductules surrounded by fibrous tissue. (Hematoxylin & eosin, ×160.)

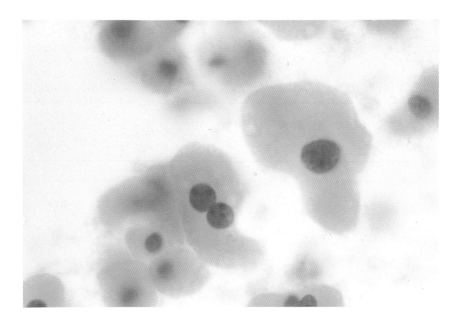

FIGURE 4–4 Normal hepatocytes with one or two central round nuclei and abundant granular cytoplasm. Nucleoli are visible. (Papanicolaou, ×250.)

or round to oval in shape with usually one or occasionally two small, round, centrally located nuclei with visible and sometimes conspicuous nucleoli and abundant granular, eosinophilic cytoplasm (Figure 4–4). Although more commonly associated with neoplastic hepatocytes, particularly hepatocellular carcinoma, cytoplasmic intranuclear invaginations may occasionally be seen in the benign cell (Figure 4–5). There is great variation in nuclear size within the normal liver, both between individuals and with increasing age.[2] Occasionally large, "atypical" cells (Figure 4–6) are present in otherwise normal-appearing groups of hepatocytes and are considered within the realm of normal. Rarely, endothelium may be present partially around groups of benign hepatocytes, but the trabeculae are still thin, not thick as in carcinoma. Subtle cellular changes may be present in cases of hepa-

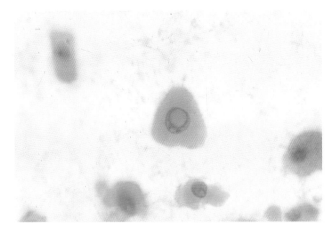

FIGURE 4–5 Normal hepatocyte with cytoplasmic intranuclear invagination. (Papanicolaou, ×250.)

FIGURE 4–6 Monolayered sheet of hepatocytes within the realm of normal. The more prominent nucleoli and the occasional "atypical" enlarged nucleus is not significant. The nuclei are round and central and maintain a low nuclear to cytoplasmic ratio even in the "atypical" cell. Note the irregular jagged outline of the group lacking an endothelial wrapping. These features help to distinguish benign groups from hepatocellular carcinoma. (Papanicolaou, ×250.)

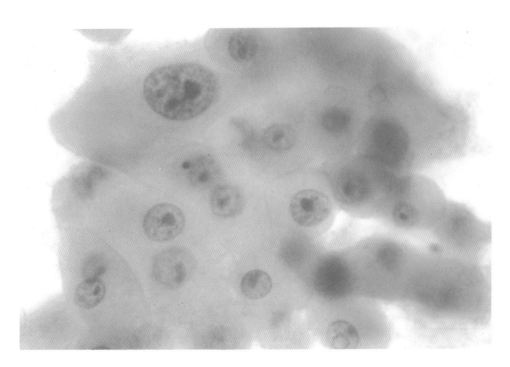

tocellular carcinoma, but it is the smear pattern of the cellular groups and the presence or absence of endothelial cells either wrapping around cell clusters or transgressing loosely cohesive sheets of hepatocytes that we find most helpful in differentiating benign hepatocytes from well-differentiated hepatocellular carcinoma[3] (see Chapter 6). Naked or stripped hepatocyte nuclei (Figure 4–7) may be present and are due to smearing and fixation artifact.[4] These nuclei should not be confused with a small cell or poorly differentiated carcinoma.

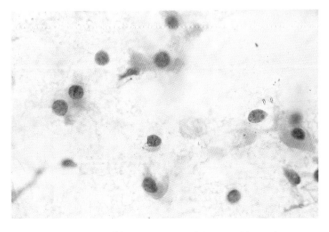

FIGURE 4–7 Stripped hepatocyte nuclei, an artifact of preparation. (Papanicolaou, ×250.)

BILE DUCT EPITHELIUM

Bile duct epithelial cells are smaller than hepatocytes (Figure 4–8) and are most commonly from the larger bile ducts lined by tall columnar, nonciliated epithelial cells. They occur mostly as monolayered sheets or aggregates and often demonstrate the classic honeycomb pattern of glandular cells (Figure 4–9). When on edge, a palisading arrangement is present (Figure 4–10), and they may rarely be seen as small tubules recapitulating their form in the portal tract (Figure 4–11). The cells are columnar with round to oval nuclei, even chromatin, and inconspicuous nucleoli. Nuclear crowding and overlapping (except in folds) should not occur in normal ductal epithelium.

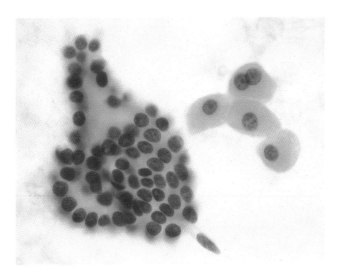

FIGURE 4–8 Benign hepatocytes (*lower right*) and bile duct epithelium (*center and left*). The bile duct cells are smaller than hepatocytes and typically occur in groups rather than singly. The nuclei are small and round and have fine, even chromatin, inconspicuous nucleoli, and are eccentrically located in a delicate cytoplasm. (Papanicolaou, ×250.)

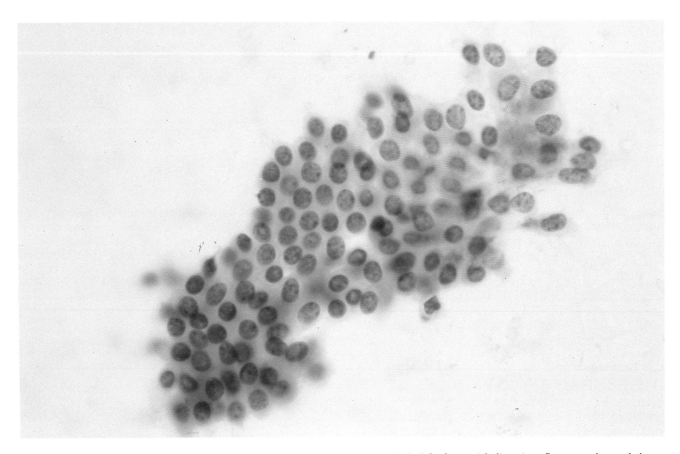

FIGURE 4–9 Bile duct epithelium in a flat, monolayered sheet with the typical glandular honeycomb pattern. (Papanicolaou, ×160.)

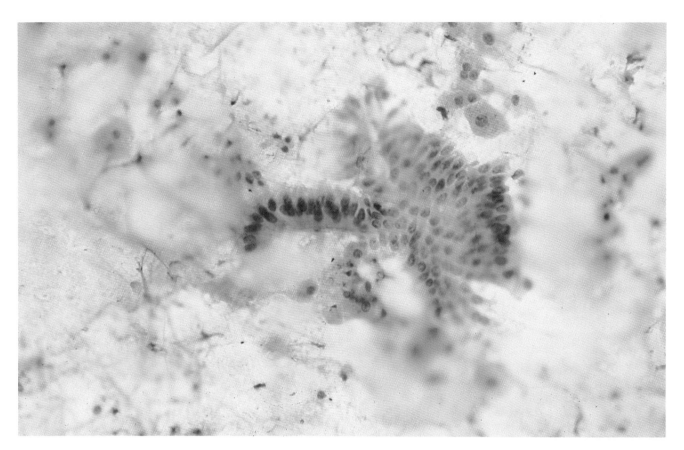

FIGURE 4–10 Bile duct epithelium with palisading "picket fence" arrangement. (Papanicolaou, ×100.)

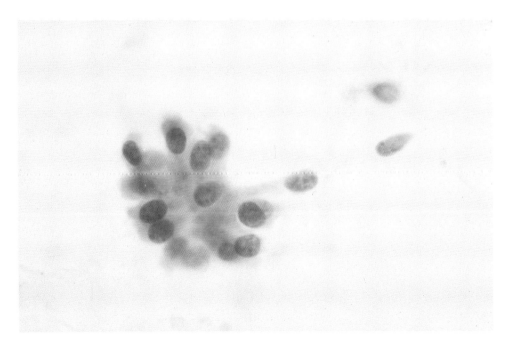

FIGURE 4–11 Bile duct epithelium forming a small acinus and recapitulating its shape in the portal tract. (Papanicolaou, ×250.)

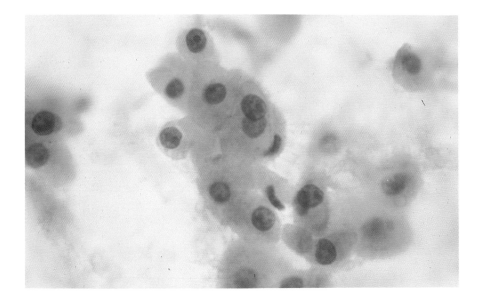

FIGURE 4–12 Normal hepatocytes with rarely observed kupffer cells wrapping around the right side of the central group of hepatocytes. The kupffer cells have a flattened, bean-shaped nucleus and distinct cytoplasm. (Papanicolaou, ×250.)

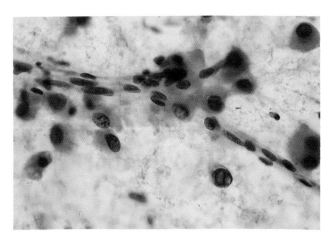

FIGURE 4–13 Endothelial cells transgressing loosely cohesive groups of hepatocytes in a well-differentiated hepatocellular carcinoma. Their nuclei are oblong with round ends and have fine, even chromatin. (Papanicolaou, ×160.)

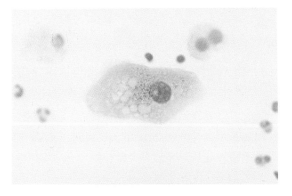

FIGURE 4–14 Lipofuscin pigment is generally present around the nucleus as uniform golden granules. This pigment is known as "wear and tear" pigment and results from the accumulation of undigested membrane material in lysosomes. (Papanicolaou, ×250.)

KUPFFER CELLS

Kupffer cells of the reticuloendothelial system are rarely appreciated in aspirates of the liver. They, along with endothelial cells, line the sinusoids separating trabeculae of hepatic parenchyma. They have a bean-shaped nucleus and distinct cytoplasm and occur singly or attached to hepatocytes (Figure 4–12).

ENDOTHELIAL CELLS

Endothelial cells are abundant in the liver as lining cells of the sinusoids but are not a prominent component of the normal liver aspirate. They may rarely be noted partially wrapping around occasional thin trabeculae of normal liver but are more often seen proliferating in a transgressing manner among loosely cohesive hepatocytes or wrapped around nests and trabeculae of hepatocellular carcinoma (Figure 4–13). The nuclei are oblong with rounded ends and have fine, evenly dispersed chromatin. The cytoplasm is bipolar and usually ill-defined.

PIGMENTS

Lipofuscin

Lipofuscin pigment, or "wear and tear" pigment, results from the accumulation of undigested membrane material in lysosomes. It is typically concentrated around the nucleus and has a golden, granular appearance (Figure 4–14).

Bile Pigment

Bile pigment varies considerably in color, texture, size, and density but is commonly present as coarse, irregular, globular clumps of green pigment (Figure 4–15). This appearance contrasts nicely with the coarse, golden granularity of lipofuscin pigment (Figure 4–16). Occasionally, with large duct obstruction, cohesive groups of hepatocytes will demonstrate cannilicular bile stasis (Figure 4–17).

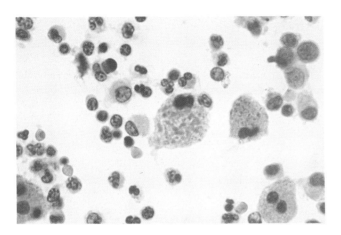

FIGURE 4–15 Bile pigment. Intracytoplasmic bile pigment varies in color, texture, size, and density but is commonly present as green, coarse, irregular clumps diffusely dispersed throughout the cytoplasm or concentrated around the periphery of the cell. (Papanicolaou, ×250.)

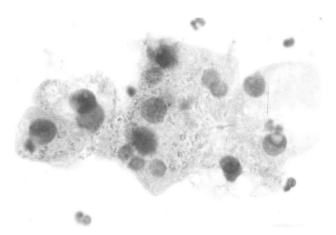

FIGURE 4–16. Lipofuscin and bile pigment. Note the golden color and coarse granularity of the lipofuscin pigment and the clumpy, globular nature of the green bile pigment. (Papanicolaou, ×250.)

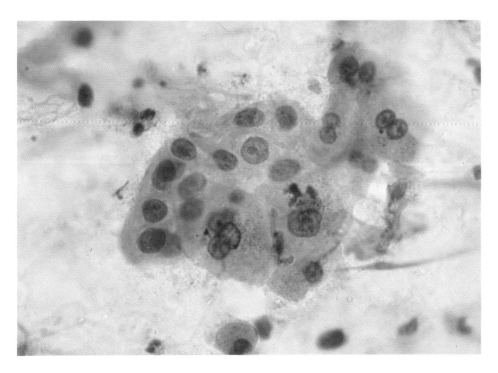

FIGURE 4–17 Cholestasis. Bile pigment is occasionally seen filling the cannilicular spaces between hepatocytes in cohesive groups and is an indication of extrahepatic obstruction. Note the columnar bile duct epithelial cells at the edge of the central hepatocytes. (Papanicolaou, ×250.)

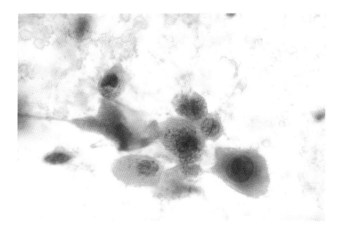

FIGURE 4–18 Iron pigment. Hemosiderin is an uncommon pigment in the liver. It is peripheral or diffuse depending on the iron load and is present as *refractile* brown-black granules on Papanicolaou stain. The iron load is heavy in this case of hemochromatosis. (Papanicolaou, ×250.)

Hemosiderin

Hemosiderin or iron pigment is not commonly seen in liver aspirates. The pigment is brown-black and refractile on Papanicolaou (Pap) stain (Figure 4–18), and depending on the iron load, will be peripheral or diffusely scattered throughout the cytoplasm.

CONTAMINANTS

The most common contaminant of the liver aspirate is mesothelium picked up from the peritoneum. These cells are easily recognizable as large, flat, monolayered sheets with evenly spaced, polygonal cells separated by clear spaces referred to as "windows" (Figure 4–19). These "windows" help differentiate these sheets of cells from bile duct epithelium. Occasionally, skeletal muscle and squamous epithelium from the skin are also seen.

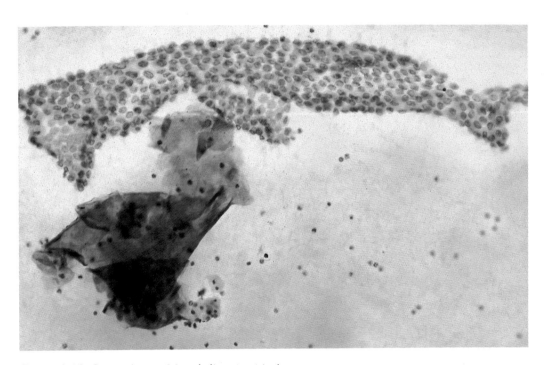

FIGURE 4–19 Contaminants. Mesothelium (*top*) is the most common contaminant from the peritoneum. It is usually present as cohesive, monolayered sheets with evenly spaced polygonal cells separated by clear "windows." (Papanicolaou, ×100.)

REFERENCES

1. Rappaport AM. The structural and functional unit of the human liver (liver acinus). Microvasc Res 1973;6:212.

2. Koss GL, Woyke S, Olszewski W. Aspiration biopsy: cytologic interpretation and histologic bases. New York: Agaku-Shoin, 1984;351.

3. Pitman MB, Szyfelbein WM. The significance of endothelium in the diagnosis of hepatocellular carcinoma. Diagn Cytopathol (in press).

4. Tao L-C. Transabdominal fine-needle aspiration biopsy. New York: Agaku-Shoin, 1990;46.

CHAPTER 5

Benign Liver Disorders

Martha Bishop Pitman and
Wanda Maria Szyfelbein

Fine needle aspiration biopsies (FNABs) of the liver are generally performed to confirm the diagnosis of a suspected neoplasm or to stage the condition of a patient with a known primary tumor. Although they are typically not performed to confirm or diagnose cirrhosis and hepatitis, (histology is necessary for an accurate diagnosis of these entities), these entities are occasionally encountered on FNAB of the liver when these processes present as a mass—for example, a regenerative nodule in cirrhosis mimicking hepatocellular carcinoma. Biopsies are also performed to confirm a benign lesion such as a simple cyst, adenoma, or abscess.

In most cases, the cytomorphologic findings of non-neoplastic and benign neoplastic lesions on aspirate alone are nonspecific, and close correlation with clinical history and other ancillary studies is necessary to confirm a suspected cytologic diagnosis. Cell block preparations of needle rinsings and core biopsies are often extremely helpful in making a definite diagnosis.

NON-NEOPLASTIC

Fatty Change

Fatty change is a nonspecific finding, and whether diffuse or focal, it can produce images on computed tomography (CT) that mimic metastatic disease.[1] One of the most common causes of fatty change in the United States is alcohol abuse; others include obesity, diabetes, and malnutrition. Fatty change can also occur as an acute response to toxic injury such as from drugs. The etiology of fatty change cannot be determined by cytomorphology alone. Fat is present in the cytoplasm of hepatocytes as large single vacuoles (macrovesicular steatosis; Figure 5–1) or as multiple small vacuoles (microvesicular steatosis; Figure 5–2).

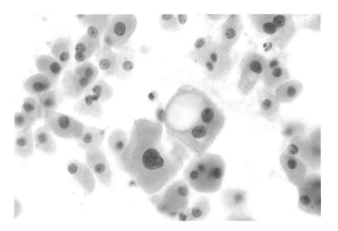

FIGURE 5–1 Macrovesicular steatosis. Benign hepatocyte with single large intracytoplasmic vacuole. (Papanicolaou, ×160.)

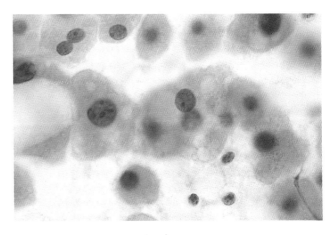

FIGURE 5–2 Microvesicular steatosis. Benign hepatocytes with multiple small intracytoplasmic vacuoles. (Papanicolaou, ×250.)

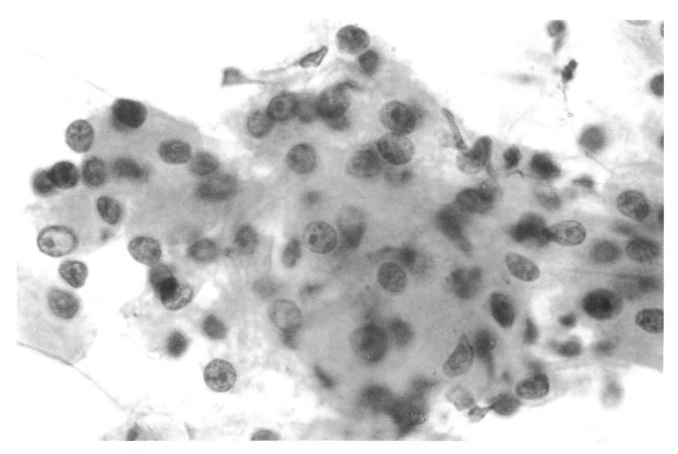

FIGURE 5–3 Cluster of reactive hepatocytes with jagged, irregular edges and no transgressing or peripheral endothelium. (Papanicolaou, ×160.)

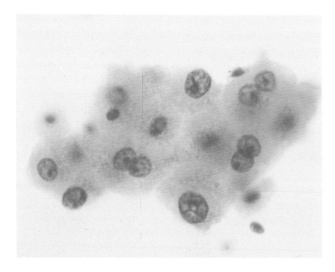

FIGURE 5–4 Reactive hepatocytes demonstrate slight nuclear pleomorphism with maintenance of low nuclear to cytoplasmic ratio, prominent nucleoli, increased numbers of binucleated hepatocytes, and bile stasis. (Papanicolaou, ×250.)

Hepatitis and Cirrhosis

Hepatitis and cirrhosis can be suggested but rarely definitively diagnosed on aspirate smears alone of FNABs of the liver.[2] These diseases often occur together and share cytomorphologic features. Reactive hepatocytes, fibrosis, and inflammation are the key common findings in these disease pro-cesses. Reactive hepatocytes occur in cohesive fragments that may be thick and multicellular, but in contrast to hepatocellular carcinoma, which at least focally forms smooth-edged trabeculae and nests often surrounded by endothelium, fragments of reactive hepatocytes typically have irregular, jagged edges without endothelial wrapping (Figure 5–3). Reactivity is also manifested by cellular and nuclear enlargement with preservation of a low nuclear to cytoplasmic (N/C) ratio, multinucleation (most commonly binucleation), cellular and nuclear pleomorphism, intranuclear pseudo-inclusions, and prominent nucleoli. Bile stasis may be evident (Figure 5–4).

Dysplastic Hepatocytes

Dysplastic hepatocytes are not an uncommon finding in reactive processes (Figure 5–5). These cells show marked cellular atypia with nuclear hyperchromasia, nuclear envelope irregularities, pleomorphism, and occasional macronucleoli. These dysplastic cells also have

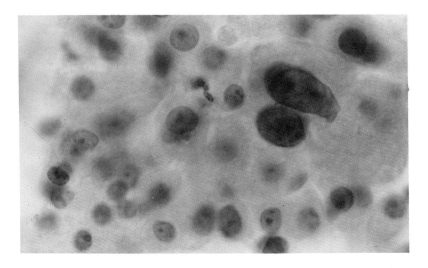

FIGURE 5–5 Dysplastic hepatocytes in the background of reactive hepatocytes. Despite the large, very pleomorphic nuclei with hyperchromasia and prominent nucleoli, the dysplastic hepatocytes maintain a low nuclear to cytoplasmic ratio and are present conspicuously among a background of reactive hepatocytes. (Papanicolaou, ×250.)

abundant cytoplasm and, thus, a low N/C ratio, and are scattered among reactive and normal hepatocytes, a key to their identity as dysplastic rather than neoplastic.[3]

Councilman Body

A councilman body or acidophil body is a necrotic hepatocyte (Figure 5–6) and is an indication of acute hepatic injury.[4,5] It is a nonspecific finding and does not indicate the nature of the injury.

Chronic Hepatitis

Chronic hepatitis implies a viral hepatitis of at least 6 months' duration. This diagnosis is suggested by the presence of a marked mononuclear cell infiltrate identified in the background of the smear and within reactive cell clusters (Figure 5–7). Active versus persistent hepatitis cannot be determined on the basis of cytology; histology is required.

FIGURE 5–6 Necrotic hepatocyte (councilman body) in a background of acute and chronic inflammation, features consistent with acute hepatic injury. (Papanicolaou, ×250.)

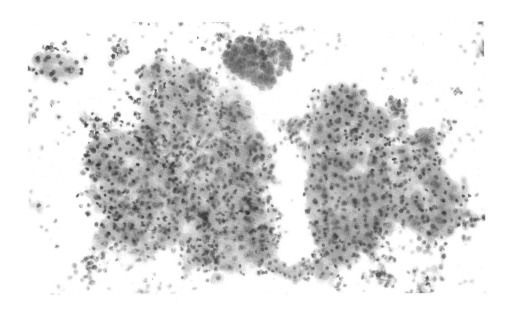

FIGURE 5–7 Clusters of reactive hepatocytes with numerous lymphocytes embedded within the clusters of reactive hepatocytes and in the background of the smear. Note the cluster of benign bile duct epithelium in the top center of the picture. (Papanicolaou, ×64.)

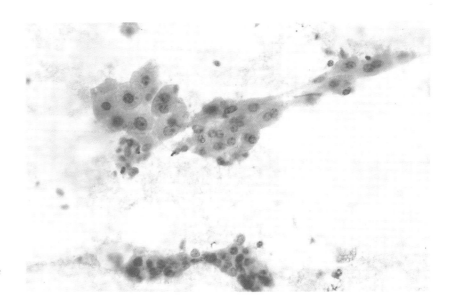

FIGURE 5–8 Cirrhosis. Two groups of reactive ductal cells associated with reactive hepatocytes. (Papanicolaou, ×250.)

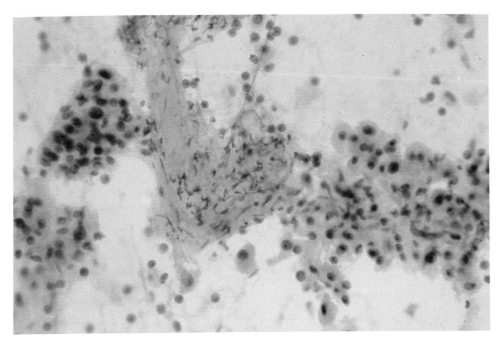

FIGURE 5–9 Cirrhosis. Reactive hepatocytes adjacent to a thick fragment of fibrous tissue. (Papanicolaou, ×100.)

Cirrhosis

Cirrhosis, by definition, requires histologic architecture to demonstrate a disorganized lobular architecture with fibrosis. Although nonspecific, these changes can be appreciated on smears of aspirates from cirrhotic livers. The key findings include reactive hepatocytes with an increased number of often atypical bile duct epithelial cells (Figure 5–8) and fibrosis (Figure 5–9). The presence of increased fibrous tissue and lymphocytes often results in crush and smear artifact (Figure 5–10). Note the irregular, jagged edges of the groups of reactive hepatocytes and the absence of either transgressing or periph-erally wrapping endothelium. These features in addition to the "irregular" atypia of the hepatocytes punctuated by dysplastic hepatocytes help in identifying these cells as benign. Tissue fragments processed as a cell block are extremely helpful in providing material for special stains and often provide just enough additional information to make a definitive diagnosis of cirrhosis (Figure 5–11) and/or chronic active hepatitis (Figure 5–12). In most cases, the radiologic picture and clinical history are already consistent with a diagnosis of cirrhosis, and an FNAB is being performed to differentiate a large regenerative nodule from early hepatocellular carcinoma (see Chapter 6).

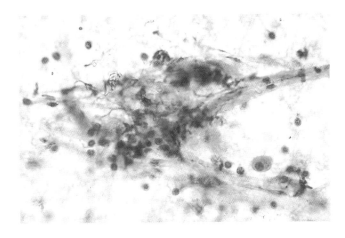

FIGURE 5–10 Crush and smear artifact of fibrous tissue and lymphoctyes in a patient with cirrhosis and chronic active hepatitis. (Papanicolaou, ×160.)

FIGURE 5–11 Cirrhosis. Cell block preparation of tissue fragments demonstrating increased fibrosis. (Trichrome, ×250.)

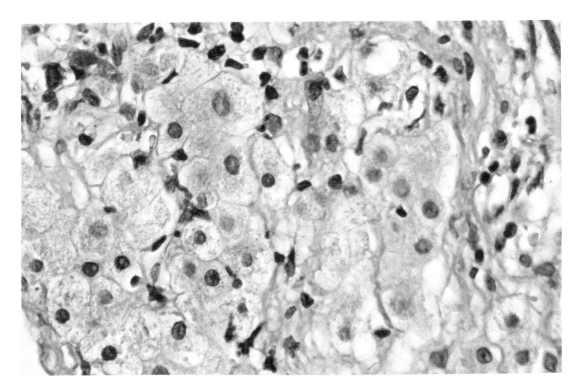

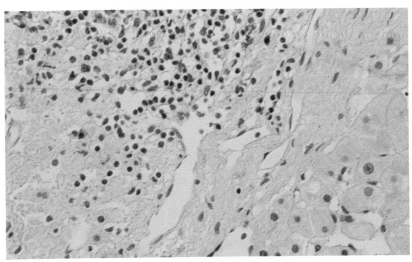

FIGURE 5–12 Chronic active hepatitis. Cell block preparation of tiny tissue fragments demonstrating infiltration of lymphocytes beyond the limiting plate of the portal tract. (Hematoxlyin & eosin, ×160.)

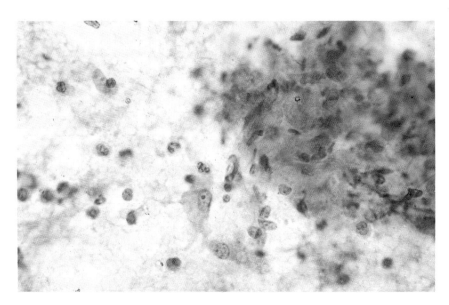

FIGURE 5–13 Granulomatous hepatitis. Aggregate of epithelioid histiocytes consistent with granuloma present in a background of inflammation. (Papanicolaou, ×160.)

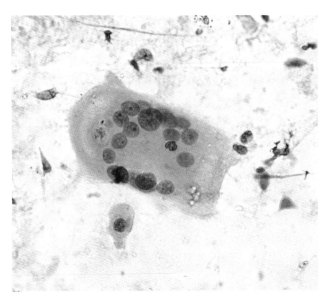

FIGURE 5–14 Granulomatous hepatitis. Langhans' type multinucleated giant cell. (Papanicolaou, ×250.)

Granulomatous Hepatitis

Granulomatous hepatitis can be identified but is usually not otherwise defined by FNAB. Clinical correlation is usually necessary to determine the causative agent. The wide range of etiologies includes infectious agents such as tuberculosis (TB) and histoplasmosis, neoplasms such as Hodgkin's disease and liver cell adenoma, hypersensitivity reactions from drugs such as sulfasalazine and phenytoin, and other conditions such as sarcoidosis and primary biliary cirrhosis.[5] The general cytologic picture of granulomatous changes is relatively uniform with common denominator findings of epithelioid cells and multinucleated giant cells, plus or minus necrotic material.[6] Epithelioid histiocytes may form loose or tightly cohesive clusters (granulomas) that may be associated with inflammatory cells (Figure 5–13) and Langhans' type multinucleated giant cells (Figure 5–14). The presence of abundant caseous-type necrosis is suggestive of TB, and an acid-fast stain should be performed; eosinophils are suggestive of drugs or Hodgkin's disease.[7] Tight, cohesive, uniformly sized granulomas without necrosis are suggestive of sarcoidosis. Without the direct identification of specific organisms, clinical correlation and other studies such as cultures are necessary to determine the etiology.

Hemochromatosis

Idiopathic hemochromatosis is an autosomal recessive disorder resulting in massive iron deposition in multiple organs including the liver. This excess in iron storage leads to parenchymal cell damage and ultimately cirrhosis. Hepatocellular carcinoma complicates 15 to 30 percent of cases.[8] On aspiration cytology, a marked increase in cytoplasmic pigment of benign hepatocytes is noted on either a Papanicolaou (Pap) stain (Figure 5–15) or a hematoxylin and eosin (H & E) stain (Figure 5–16), where the granules appear golden and refractile. Iron deposits may also be visible in the bile duct epithelium and stroma, but only in kupffer cells present in areas of parenchymal necrosis.[5] Marked reactive hepatocyte atypia may be present (Figure 5–17), and careful attention must be paid to rule out the presence of hepatocellular carcinoma. One helpful feature is the inability of malignant hepatocytes to store iron[9] and thus the lack of iron deposition in these cells (Figures 5–18 and 5–19).

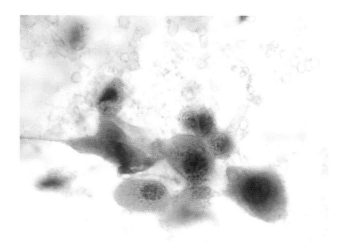

FIGURE 5–15 Hemochromatosis. Benign hepatocytes with abundant golden, granular, refractile iron pigment deposits. (Papanicolaou, ×250.)

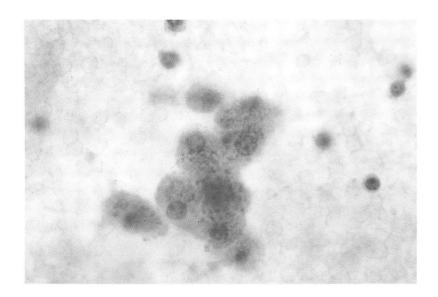

FIGURE 5–16 Hemochromatosis. Benign hepatocytes with abundant golden, granular, refractile iron pigment deposits. (Hematoxylin & eosin, ×250.)

FIGURE 5–17 Hemochromatosis. Marked reactive hepatocyte atypia is often associated with this disease due to the parenchymal damage, regeneration, and ultimate cirrhosis that results. The presence of iron deposition in the cytoplasm supports a reactive diagnosis as malignant hepatocytes cannot store iron. (Hematoxylin & eosin, ×250.)

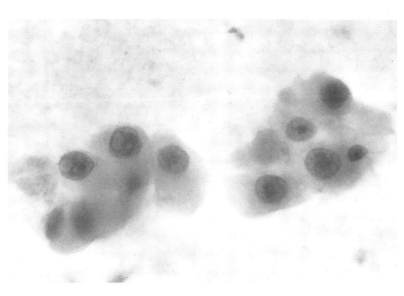

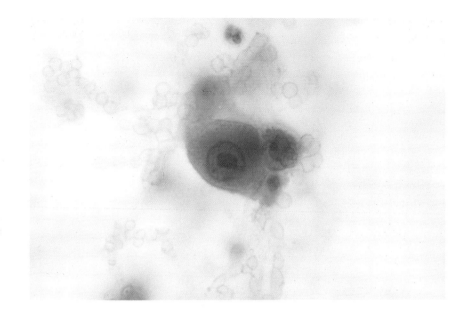

FIGURE 5–18 Hepatocellular carcinoma associated with hemochromatosis. Note the presence of iron pigment in the benign hepatocyte on the left and the lack of pigment in the malignant cell on the right. (Hematoxylin & eosin, ×250.)

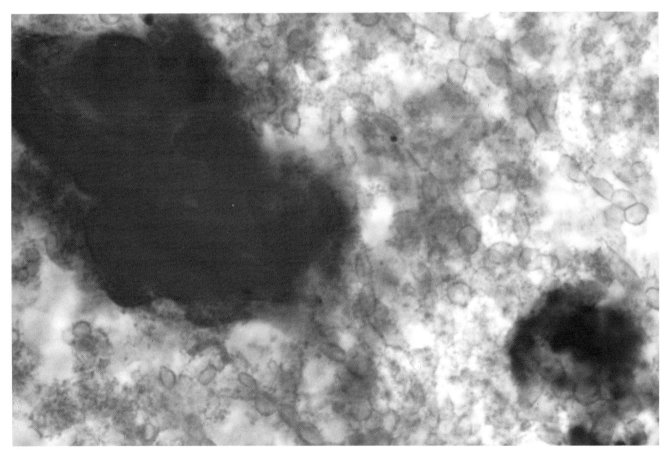

FIGURE 5–19 Hepatocellular carcinoma associated with hemochromatosis. This iron stain clearly differentiates the benign reactive (blue-staining) hepatocytes from the group of hepatocellular carcinoma cells lacking pigment. (Prussian blue, ×250.)

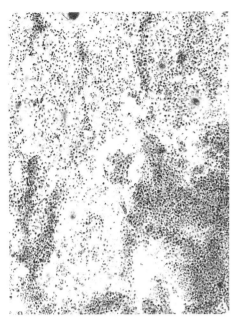
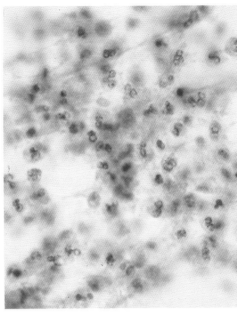

FIGURE 5–20 Abscess. Aspirated material consists almost entirely of polymorphonuclear leukocytes. Necrotic hepatocytes are rarely appreciated. (Papanicolaou; left ×40, right ×250.)

Pyogenic Abscess

Pyogenic abscess is the most common type of liver abscess.[7] Imaging techniques are generally very accurate in detecting visceral abscesses,[10] which may be single or multiple. Percutaneous aspirations are performed for tissue confirmation, culture, and drainage. Cultures are positive in up to 80 percent of cases.[6] The aspirated material looks like pus, is foul smelling, and microscopically is composed of a sea of neutrophils in a background of debris usually without obvious necrotic hepatocytes (Figure 5–20). Organisms are rarely identified on Gram's stain.

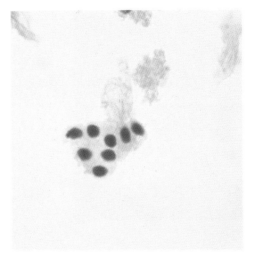

FIGURE 5–21 Simple cyst. Small cluster of cuboidal lining epithelial cells. (Papanicolaou, ×250.)

Simple Cyst

Solitary, unilocular intrahepatic cysts are typically asymptomatic but may present as a mass.[11] They are of variable size and are lined by flattened to cuboidal epithelium (Figure 5–21). The intracystic fluid may be serous or mucoid and even bloody with trauma. A superimposed infection results in a purulent fluid. Cystic debris typical of any cyst should be evident on the cytology preparation (Figure 5–22).

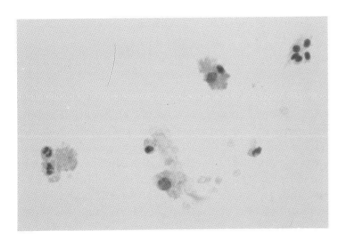

FIGURE 5–22 Simple cyst. Cystic debris typical of any cyst with degenerated lining and inflammatory cells. (Papanicolaou, ×250.)

Hydatid Cyst

Hydatid cysts, most commonly caused by the dog tapeworm *Echinococcus granulosus*, are large, unilocular cysts filled with daughter cysts collectively known as hydatid sand (Figure 5–23). The presence of a hydatid cyst is considered by some to be an absolute contraindication to FNAB due to the risk of rupture and potential for anaphylactic shock;[12] however, radiologic identification is not absolutely specific,[13] and biopsies of such lesions do not always have complications.[14] Diagnostic findings after aspiration include a thick, pasty, yellow-brown ("anchovy paste") material that microscopically contains scoleces with hooklets that stain positively with a modified acid-fast stain (Figure 5–24).

central stellate scar is the *sine qua non* of FNH and is the distinguishing diagnostic feature in differentiating FNH from liver cell adenoma. On FNA aspirate smears alone this distinction may be impossible to see. The hepatocytes in both FNH and adenoma are normal, benign hepatocytes (Figures 5–27 and 5–28). The presence of fibrous tissue fragments and bile duct epithelium help to rule out adenoma but are often not present; their presence introduces cirrhosis into the differential diagnosis. The spectrum of reactive and dysplastic hepatocytes typical of cirrhosis should not be present in the aspirate of FNH. The features that distinguish FNH from well-differentiated hepatocellular carcinoma include the uniform benignity of the hepatocytes with low N/C ratio, small round nuclei without prominent nucleoli, and a

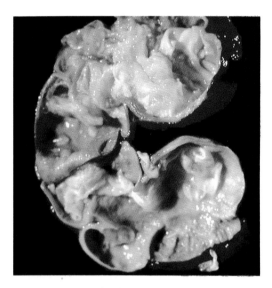

FIGURE 5–23 Hydatid (echinococcal) cyst. Large unilocular cyst filled with daughter cysts (hydatid sand).

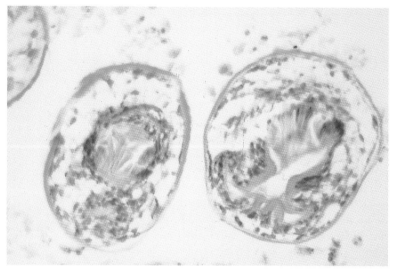

FIGURE 5–24 Echinococcal scoleces in cross-section demonstrating central hooklets that stain red with a modified acid-fast stain. (Modified Ziehl-Neelsen, ×250.)

Focal Nodular Hyperplasia

Focal nodular hyperplasia (FNH) is considered by most to be a hamartomatous, developmental defect rather than a true neoplasm.[15] As it is an asymptomatic process in the majority of patients, FNH is usually diagnosed during a celiotomy or other diagnostic procedures.[16] On magnetic resonance imaging scan (Figure 5–25), the tumor may appear isointense without contrast and may or may not illustrate the classic central scar. Grossly FNH is a lobulated mass as opposed to the solitary nodule seen in liver cell adenoma (Figure 5–26). The

smear pattern composed typically of large flat sheets with irregular, jagged edges lacking both peripheral and transgressing endothelium. If tissue fragments or a core biopsy is obtained for cell block, a definitive diagnosis can often be made. The presence of thick, fibrous vascular bands separating aggregates of benign hepatocytes is support- ive of a diagnosis of FNH[17] (Figures 5–29 and 5–30). Correlation of aspirate findings with radiographic findings and clinical history is imperative in making an accurate diagnosis.

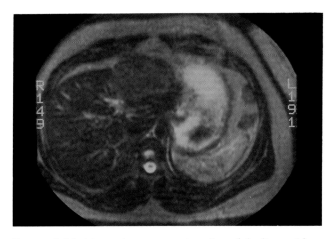

FIGURE 5–25 Magnetic resonance imaging of the liver with focal nodular hyperplasia. The tumor in the left lobe of the liver is an isointense mass. (Courtesy of Dr. Giles Boland, Masschusetts General Hospital, Boston.)

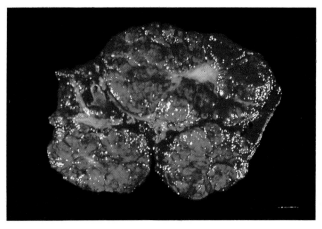

FIGURE 5–26 Gross focal nodular hyperplasia. The tumor is multilobulated and contains the typical central stellate scar in the upper, largest nodule.

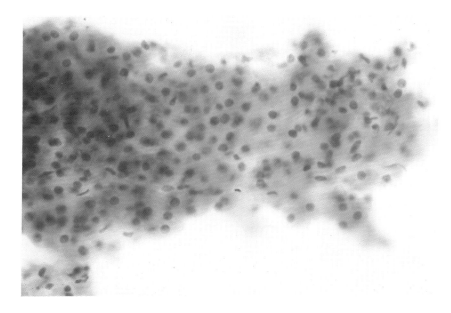

FIGURE 5–27 Focal nodular hyperplasia. Cluster of benign hepatocytes with uniform nuclear features. Note the irregular edges and the lack of either peripheral or transgressing endothelium. (Papanicolaou, ×100.)

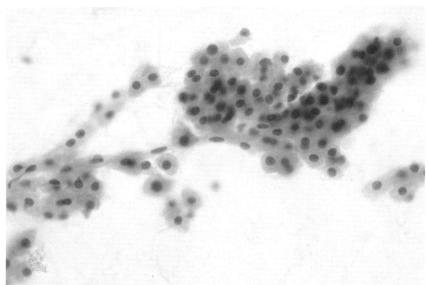

FIGURE 5–28 Focal nodular hyperplasia. Nonspecific benign hepatocytes. (Papanicolaou, ×100.)

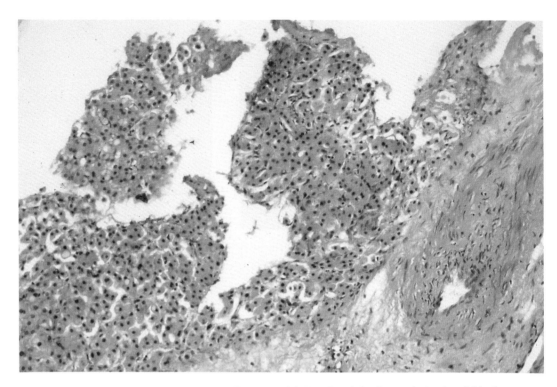

FIGURE 5–29 Focal nodular hyperplasia. A cell block preparation demonstrates benign hepatocytes surrounded by very
thick bands of fibrous tissue with large muscular arteries.
(Hematoxylin & eosin, ×25.)

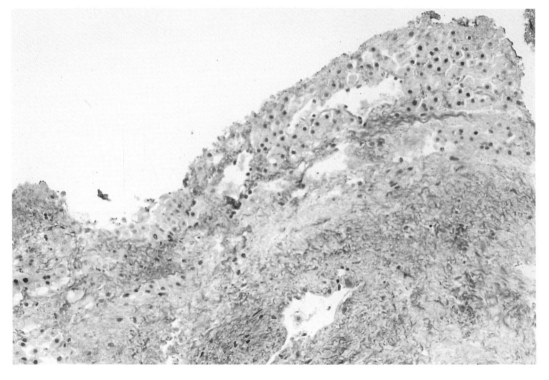

FIGURE 5–30 Focal nodular hyperplasia. A trichrome stain
illustrates the degree of fibrous tissue. (Trichrome, ×25.)

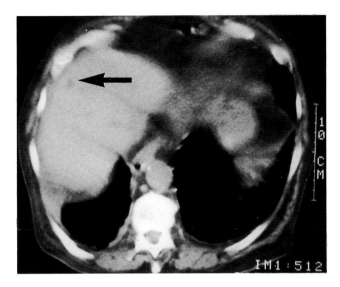

FIGURE 5–31 Bile duct hamartoma. Computed tomography demonstrates multiple nodules (*arrow*) mimicking metastatic carcinoma. (Courtesy of Dr. Giles Boland, Massachusetts General Hospital, Boston.)

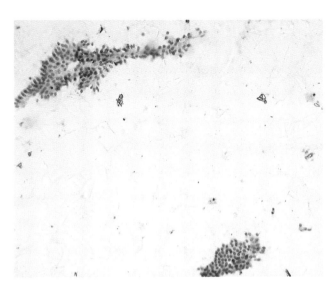

FIGURE 5–32 Bile duct hamartoma. Aspirate smears demonstrate numerous clusters of benign bile duct epithelium and scant benign hepatocytes. (Papanicolaou, ×80.)

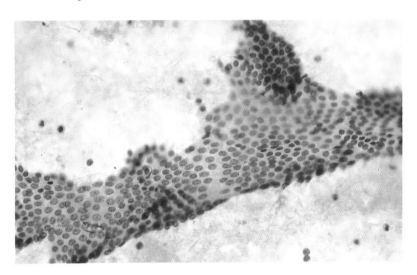

FIGURE 5–33 Bile duct hamartoma. Bile duct epithelium with the typical honeycombed pattern of glandular epithelium. No atypia is noted. (Papanicolaou, ×100.)

Bile Duct Hamartoma

Bile duct hamartoma (BDH) is an incidental finding that may be single or multiple, and may present as small nodules mimicking metastatic carcinoma on radiographic studies[18] (Figure 5–31). The lesions are typically less than 1 cm and are composed of an unencapsulated proliferation of often dilated bile ducts embedded in a dense fibrous stroma that blends into the adjacent liver. On FNAB smears, the fibrous tissue often stays behind, yielding only numerous groups of normal-appearing bile duct epithelium (Figure 5–32) with their monolayered, honeycombed appearance (Figure 5–33). Normal liver may also appear on the smear, which often leads to a "negative, normal liver components" type of diagnosis. Cell block preparations (Figure 5–34) are extremely helpful in making a definitive diagnosis in these cases.

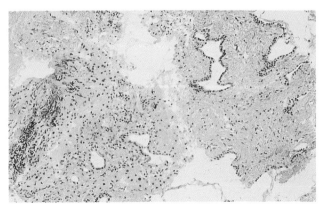

FIGURE 5–34 Bile duct hamartoma. A cell block preparation demonstrates the typical histomorphology of widely scattered, dilated bile ducts in a fibrous tissue background. (Hematoxylin & eosin, ×40.

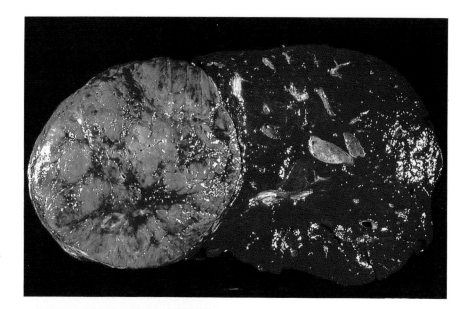

FIGURE 5–35　Liver cell adenoma. This tumor illustrates the classic features of a well-circumscribed, yellow mass with foci of hemorrhage.

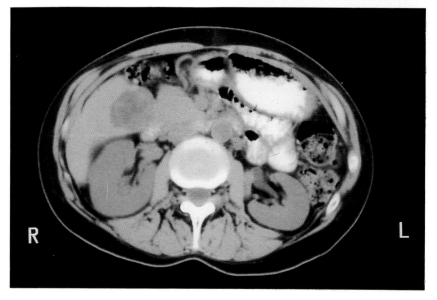

FIGURE 5–36　Liver cell adenoma. Computed tomography of the liver shows a hypodense, well-circumscribed lesion. (Courtesy of Dr. Peter Mueller, Massachusetts General Hospital, Boston)

NEOPLASTIC

Liver Cell Adenoma

Liver cell adenoma (LCA) is usually a solitary, well-circumscribed, encapsulated lesion, often with foci of hemorrhage and necrosis (Figure 5–35), that occurs most commonly in women over 30 years old who have been taking oral contraceptives for more than 5 years.[19] Compared to FNH, these tumors are more likely to hemorrhage, undergo necrosis, and rupture.[16] LCA has been reported to progress to hepatocellular carcinoma on rare occasions.[20] Adenomas on CT scan (Figure 5–36) are generally hypodense without contrast but show variable densities with contrast. Angiography reveals a hypervascular lesion with a peripheral blood supply.[16] Despite convincing historical and radiographic evidence of an adenoma, FNAB is often performed for confirma-

tion; in other cases, the clinical data may not be supportive of an adenoma, and a biopsy is performed to rule out malignancy. FNAB smears will show a single population of benign hepatocytes. Although hepatocytes in adenomas are notably larger than non-neoplastic hepatocytes on histology,[5] this feature is generally not appreciated on an isolated aspiration of adenoma alone. The most striking feature of the smears is the absence of other cellular elements, such as bile duct epithelium and fibrous tissue. This is the key to the diagnosis. The hepatocytes are arranged in small to large groups and often occur singly (Figures 5–37 and 5–38). The groups are flat with irregular edges and no peripheral or transgressing endothelium[17] (Figure 5–39). The nuclei are uniform without prominent nucleoli, and cytoplasm is abundant. The differential diagnosis is with normal liver, regenerative nodule, and FNH. Aspirates of normal liver should

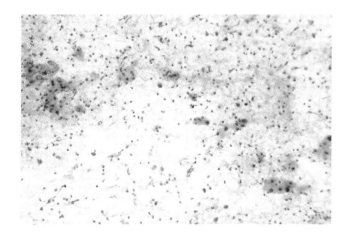

FIGURE 5–37 Liver cell adenoma. Aspirate smears show small and large clusters as well as single benign hepatocytes without the presence of fibrous tissue or bile duct epithelium. (Papanicolaou, ×40.)

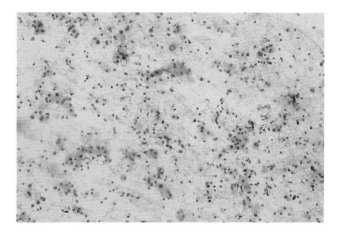

FIGURE 5–38 Liver cell adenoma. All foci of the smear will show the same monomorphic population of benign liver cells. (Papanicolaou, ×40.)

contain bile duct epithelium. The clinical presence of a mass and confirmation of the needle placement within the mass should rule out this diagnosis. A regenerative nodule should show reactive atypia and possibly fibrosis. Focal nodular hyperplasia should also have bile duct epithelium and is likely to have fibrosis on the smears. A cell block preparation showing a solid sheet of benign hepatocytes without interspersed portal tracts (Figure 5–40) is very helpful in making a definitive diagnosis. In cases where a core sample is not available or is inadequate for diagnosis, the diagnosis should indicate benign liver and a differential diagnosis should be given.

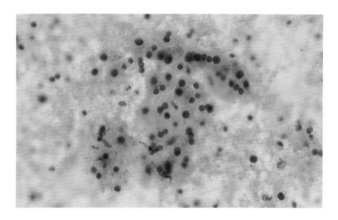

FIGURE 5–39 Liver cell adenoma. The hepatocytes are typical benign hepatocytes that may show some features of reactivity (increased numbers of binucleated cells) but no architectural or cytomorphologic features of hepatocellular carcinoma. (Papanicolaou, ×160.)

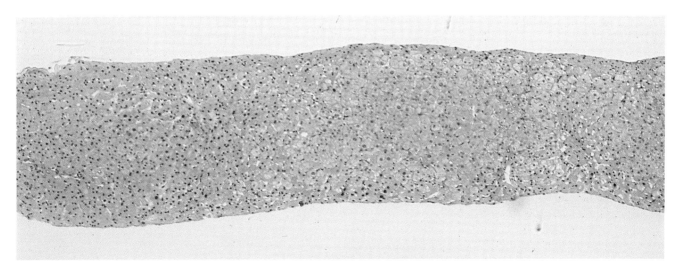

FIGURE 5–40 Liver cell adenoma. Cell block preparation of a core biopsy demonstrates a large sheet of benign hepatocytes without intervening portal triads. (Hematoxylin & eosin, ×10.)

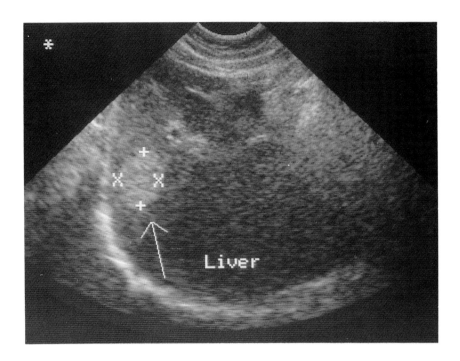

FIGURE 5–41 Cavernous hemangioma. Ultrasound of the liver demonstrates a well-demarcated, hyperechoic mass. (Courtesy of Dr. Peter Mueller, Massachusetts General Hospital, Boston.)

Cavernous Hemangioma

Cavernous hemangioma (CH) is the most common benign neoplasm of the liver, occurring more commonly in female patients under 40 but most often in elderly men.[21] They are generally less than 5 cm and occur most commonly just under the capsule. The typical ultrasound appearance of a CH is a hyperechoic mass[22] (Figure 5–41).

Fine needle aspiration biopsy is generally contraindicated for CH, but transhepatic rather than transcapsular approaches have decreased bleeding complications from FNAB of these lesions.[14] In addition, even with well-defined criteria for diagnosis using CT and angiography, not all will be identified, and an FNAB may be performed to rule out malignancy. The aspirate smears are very bloody, often yielding only scant fragments of fibrous tissue (Figure 5–42) and aggregates of benign spindle cells (endothelium) (Figure 5–43). These aspirates are often read as nondiagnostic. A cell block may be diagnostic. Dilated, endothelially lined blood-filled spaces are separated by thick fibrous septae and are well demarcated from the adjacent liver (Figures 5–44 and 5–45).

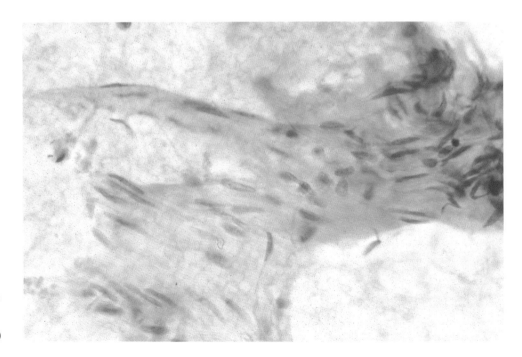

FIGURE 5–42 Cavernous hemangioma. Aspirate smears often show abundant blood with only scant fragments of mesenchymal connective tissue. (Papanicolaou, ×160.)

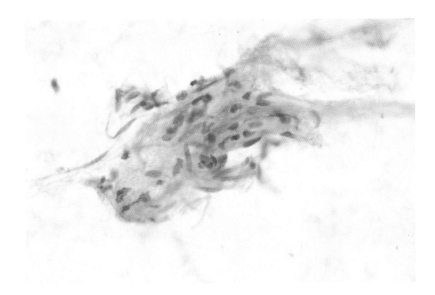

FIGURE 5–43 Cavernous hemangioma. Fragments of benign spindle cells have a loosely cohesive nature unlike the tightly cohesive fragments of fibrous tissue in cirrhosis. (Papanicolaou, ×100.)

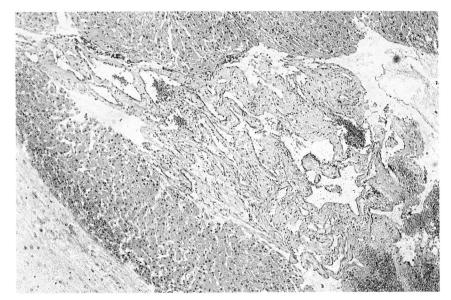

FIGURE 5–44 Cavernous hemangioma. Cell block preparation of a tissue fragment demonstrating the thick-walled septae of the vascular spaces. (Hematoxylin & eosin, ×25.)

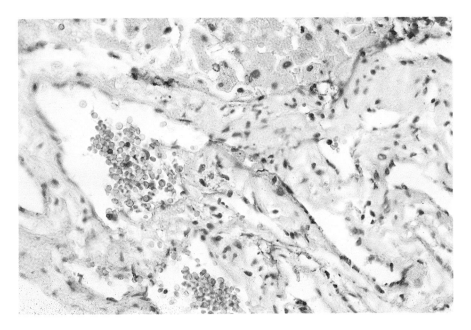

FIGURE 5–45 Cavernous hemangioma. A higher power magnification better llustrates the intraluminal red blood cells within these thick-walled spaces. (Hematoxylin & eosin, ×100.)

REFERENCES

1. Halvorsen RA, Korobkin M, Ram PC, Thompson WM. CT appearance of focal fatty infiltration of the liver. AJR Am J Roentgenol 1982;139:277–281.

2. Perry MD, Johnston WW. Needle biopsy of the liver for the diagnosis of nonneoplastic liver disease. Acta Cytol 1985;29:385–390.

3. Berman JJ, McNeill RE. Cirrhosis with atypia: a potential pitfall in the interpretation of liver aspirates. Acta Cytol 1988; 32:11–14.

4. Lundquist A, Åkerman M. Fine-needle aspiration biopsy in acute hepatitis and liver cirrhosis. Ann Clin Res 1970;2:197–203.

5. Kanel GC, Korula J. Atlas of liver pathology. Philadelphia: WB Saunders, 1992;229.

6. Stormby N, Åkerman M. Aspiration cytology in the diagnosis of granulomatous liver lesions. Acta Cytol 1973;17:200–204.

7. Tao L-C. Transabdominal fine-needle aspiration biopsy. New York: Agaku-Shoin, 1990;46.

8. Powell LW, Kerr JFR. The pathology of the liver in hemochromatosis. Pathol Annu 1975;5:317–337.

9. Frias-Hidvegi D. Guides to clinical aspiration biopsy: liver and pancreas. New York: Igaku-Shoin, 1988;72.

10. Mueller PR, Van Sonnenberg E. Interventional radiology in the chest and abdomen. N Engl J Med 1990;322:1364–1374.

11. Flagg RS, Robinson DW. Solitary nonparasitic hepatic cysts. Arch Surg 1967;95:964–973.

12. Koss LG, Woyke S, Olszewski W. Aspiration biopsy: cytologic interpretation and histologic bases. Tokyo: Igaku-Shoin, 1984;355–356.

13. Roemer CE, Ferrucci J, Mueller PR, et al. Hepatic cysts: diagnosis and therapy by sonographic needle aspiration. Am J Radiol 1981; 136:1065–1070.

14. Smith EH. Complications of percutaneous abdominal fine needle biopsy. Radiology 1991;178:253–258.

15. Robbins SL, Cotran RS, Kumar V. Pathologic basis of disease. 3rd ed. Philadelphia: WB Saunders, 1984;934.

16. Kerlin P, Davis GL, McGill DB, et al. Hepatic adenoma and focal nodular hyperplasia: clinical, pathologic and radiologic features. Gastroenterology 1983;84:994–1002.

17. Pitman MB, Szyfelbein WM. The significance of endothelium in the FNA diagnosis of hepatocellular carcinoma. Diagn. Cytopathol (in press).

18. Saló J, Concepció B, Vilella A, Ginés P, Gilabert R, Castells A, Bruguera M, Rodés J. Bile-duct hamartomas presenting as multiple focal lesions on hepatic ultrasonography. Am J Gastroenterol 1992;87:221–223.

19. Edmondson HA, Henderson B, Benton B. Liver cell adenomas associated with use of oral contraceptives. N Engl J Med 1976;294:470–472.

20. Tao L-CT. Oral contraceptive associated liver cell adenoma and hepatocellular carcinoma. Cytomporphology and mechanism of malignant transformation. Cancer 1991;68:341–347.

21. Zafrani ES. Update on vascular tumors of the liver. J Hepatol 1989;8:125–130.

22. Nichols FC, van Heerden JA, Weiland CH. Benign liver tumors. Surg Clin North Am 1989;69:297–314.

PART

III

Cytomorphology of the Malignant Aspirate

CHAPTER

6

Primary Malignant Liver Tumors

Martha Bishop Pitman and
Wanda Maria Szyfelbein

HEPATOCELLULAR CARCINOMA

Despite its relative low incidence in the United states, hepatocellular carcinoma (HCC) is the most common primary malignancy of the liver in the world, with the highest incidence in Africa and Asia.[1] It predominantly affects older men. Predisposing conditions include chronic active hepatitis B and C, alcoholic cirrhosis, hemochromatosis, toxins such as vinyl chloride and thorotrast, aflatoxins, and anabolic steroids.[1]

Most cases of HCC in the United States arise in a cirrhotic liver, making diagnosis by fine needle aspiration biopsy (FNAB) often very difficult, particularly when dealing with a small, well-differentiated tumor or small sample of a large one. Serum alpha-fetoprotein (AFP) levels may be helpful if available. In our experience, the results of an AFP test are almost never available at the time of the biopsy. Most patients with HCC will have a serum AFP level over 400 ng/ml (normal 5–10 ng/ml), but a normal level does not exclude the presence of a tumor.[2]

Hepatocellular carcinoma is known for its varied growth patterns and cytomorphologic features that not only characterize different tumors but reflect various growth patterns of the same tumor as well.[3] Several characterizations have been proposed,[4,5] but we prefer the simple subclassification of HCC as well, moderately, and poorly differentiated tumors, identifying the variants, particularly fibrolamellar HCC, as we do for histopathologic diagnoses.

Grossly, HCC is as heterogeneous in its appearance as it is in its morphology. The tumor may be present as a solitary mass that may be very small (Figure 6–1) or large, replacing most of an entire lobe (Figure 6–2); as multiple nodules mimicking metastatic malignancy (Figure 6–3); or as a diffuse process (Figure 6–4).

Well Differentiated

Well-differentiated hepatocellular carcinoma (WDHCC) is the most difficult to diagnose on FNAB. The tumor cells have obvious hepatocytic features and very subtle malignant characteristics. In our experience and that of others,[6] the arrangement of the cells on the smear is usually more helpful for making the diagnosis than the cytomorphology of individual hepatocytes. The classic presentation of WDHCC and one, which in our opinion, is absolutely diagnostic of WDHCC is illustrated in Figures 6–5 through 6–8. Aspirate smears are very cellular and composed of cohesive nests and thick trabeculae with smooth, rounded edges (Figure 6–5). Peripheral endothelial cells are apparent wrapping around these nests and trabeculae (Figure 6–6, arrow). This is *not* a feature of a benign or reactive process. A bland, rather benign appearance of the hepatocytes is noted, with cells having a slightly elevated nuclear to cytoplasmic (N/C) ratio, round to oval centrally placed nuclei, often inconspicuous nucleoli, and abundant granular cytoplasm (Figure 6–7). Although we do not routinely use air-dried May-Grünwald-Giemsa (MGG)–stained smears on our liver aspirates, these features are also apparent on this preparation (Figure 6–8).

The presence of cirrhosis or hepatitis and reactive hepatocytic features does not rule out a concomitant carcinoma. In fact, these benign changes are the very breeding ground for the development of HCC.

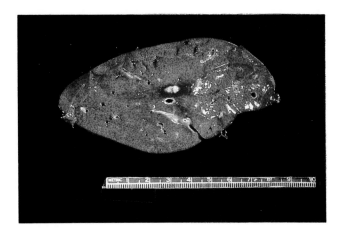

FIGURE 6–1 Hepatocellular carcinoma. Small, solitary nodule of hepatocellular carcinoma. (Courtesy of Dr. Fiona Graeme-Cook, Massachusetts General Hospital, Boston.)

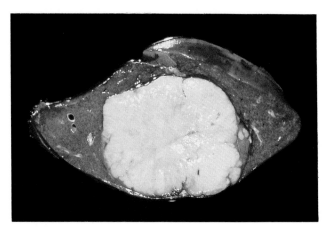

FIGURE 6–2 Hepatocellular carcinoma. Large nodule of hepatocellular carcinoma almost replacing an entire lobe. (Courtesy of Dr. Fiona Graeme-Cook, Massachusetts General Hospital, Boston.)

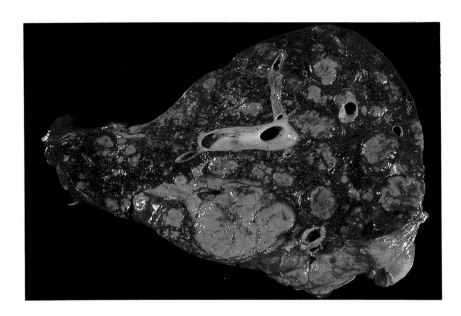

FIGURE 6–3 Hepatocellular carcinoma. Large and small scattered nodules of hepatocellular carcinoma resembling metastatic disease. (Courtesy of Dr. Carolyn Compton, Massachusetts General Hospital, Boston.)

FIGURE 6–4 Hepatocellular carcinoma. Multiple small nodules of hepatocellular carcinoma infiltrating the liver in a diffuse manner. (Courtesy of Dr. Fiona Graeme-Cook, Massachusetts General Hospital, Boston.)

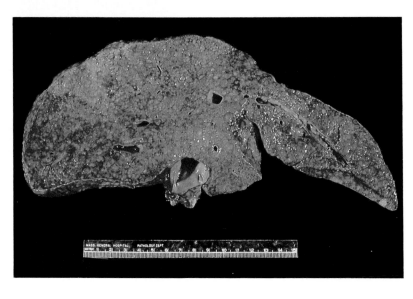

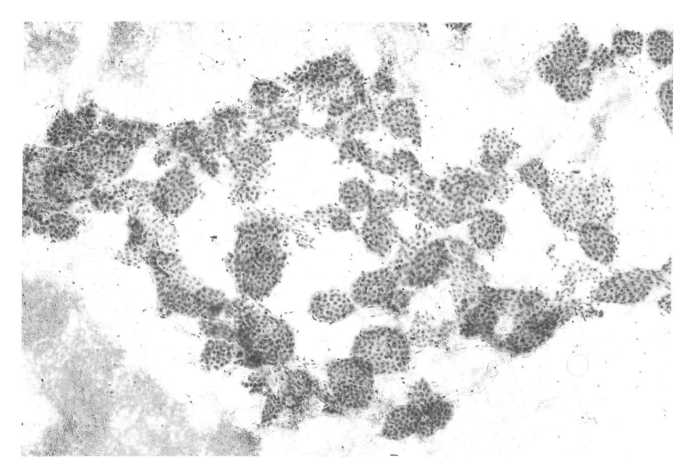

FIGURE 6–5 Well-differentiated hepatocellular carcinoma.
Classic smear pattern illustrating rounded and smooth-edged
cohesive nests and trabeculae of small uniform hepatocytes.
(Papanicolaou, ×250.)

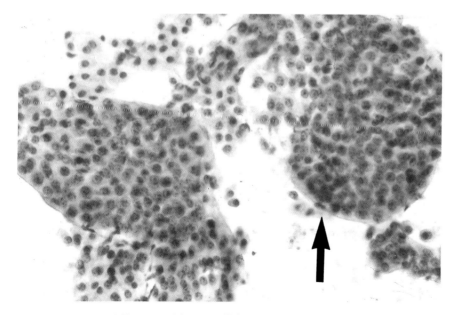

FIGURE 6–6 Well-differentiated hepatocellular carcinoma.
Endothelial cells (*arrow*) are present wrapping around
rounded cohesive nests and trabeculae of hepatocytes. (Papanicolaou, ×100.)

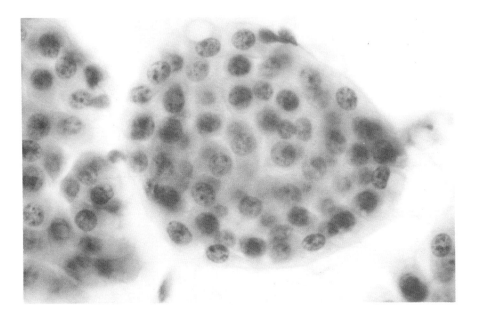

FIGURE 6–7 Well-differentiated hepatocellular carcinoma. The hepatocytes are relatively bland with a slightly elevated nuclear to cytoplasmic ratio; round, regular, centrally placed nuclei; often small inconspicuous nucleoli; and abundant granular cytoplasm. (Papanicolaou stain, ×250.)

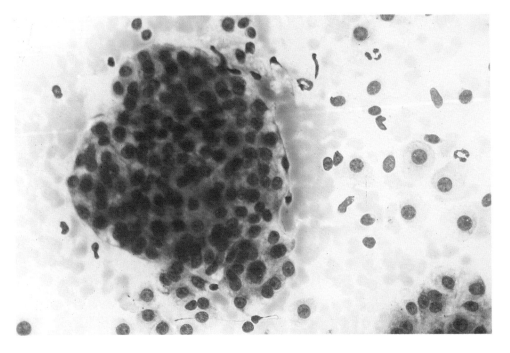

FIGURE 6–8 Well-differentiated hepatocellular carcinoma. Rounded nests of bland hepatocytes enveloped by endothelium. (May-Grünwald-Giemsa, ×100.)

Figure 6–9 and 6–10 show an aspirate of a cirrhotic liver with one prominent nodule clinically thought to be a regenerative nodule. Although other areas of the smear were representative of cirrhosis, these illustrations depict focal changes diagnostic of WDHCC. Again, notice the smear pattern of varying sized, cohesive nests and thick trabeculae (Figure 6–9) and the presence of peripherally wrapping endothelium (Figure 6–10, arrow).

In our experience, the presence of endothelium on smear preparations is an extremely important diagnostic component of HCC.[7] These endothelial cells are not consistently present peripherally wrapping around hepatocytes; they may transgress the center of loosely cohesive sheets of hepatocytes instead. The abnormal arrangement of hepatocytes in a loosely cohesive sheet that appears to be held together only by a proliferation of endothelial cells penetrating and transgressing the sheet is a common characteristic of HCC[7] (Figures 6–11 and 6–12). The hepatocytes maintain their hepatocytic features and show only slight pleomorphism and increased N/C ratio (Figure 6–13). This transgressing endothelium may rarely be found in benign reactive conditions, but when present, particularly in a prominent manner, supports the diagnosis of HCC. Supplemental cell block preparations are often very helpful in supporting a malignant diagnosis (Figure 6–14).

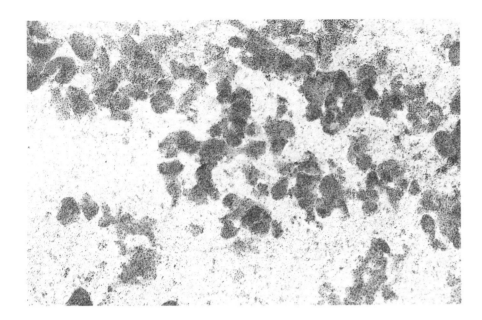

FIGURE 6–9 Well-differentiated hepatocellular carcinoma. Classic smear pattern diagnostic of hepatocellular carcinoma present in a smear that was otherwise diagnostic of cirrhosis. (Papanicolaou, ×160.)

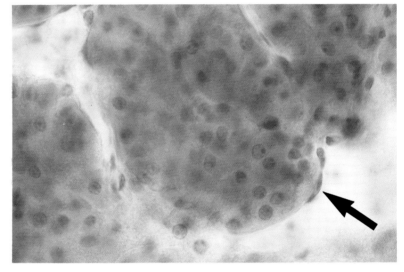

FIGURE 6–10 Well-differentiated hepatocellular carcinoma. Same slide as in Figure 6–9 at higher magnification illustrating the peripherally wrapping endothelial cells (*arrow*). (Papanicolaou, ×100.)

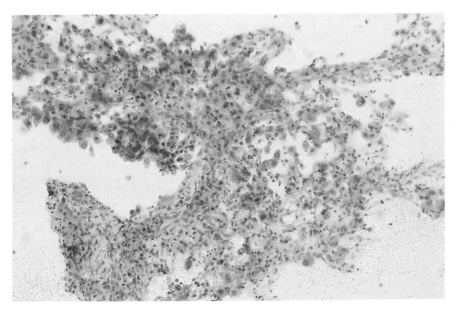

FIGURE 6–11 Well-differentiated hepatocellular carcinoma. Flat dishesive sheet of hepatocytes transgressed by proliferating band of endothelium. (Papanicolaou, ×160.)

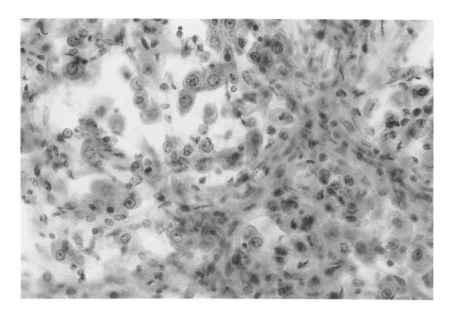

FIGURE 6–12 Well-differentiated hepato-cellular carcinoma. Same slide as in Figure 6–11 at higher magnification illustrating a dishesive sheet of hepatocytes with a slightly increased nuclear to cytoplasmic ratio and round, central, bland nuclei, transgressed by proliferating endothelium characteristic of hepatocellular carcinoma. (Papanicolaou, ×160.)

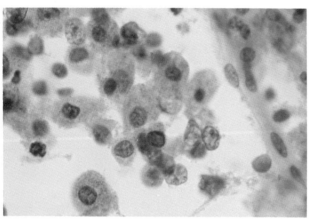

FIGURE 6–13 Well-differentiated hepatocellular carcinoma. Hepatocytes with a slightly increased nuclear to cytoplasmic ratio and mild nuclear atypia. (Papanicolaou, ×250.)

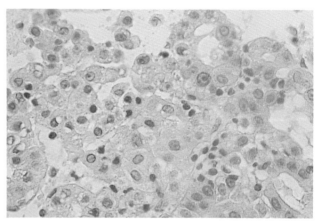

FIGURE 6–14 Well-differentiated hepatocellular carcinoma. Cell block preparation showing acinar formation by bland hepatocytes, an architectural abnormality often seen in hepatocellular carcinoma. (Hematoxylin & eosin, ×160.)

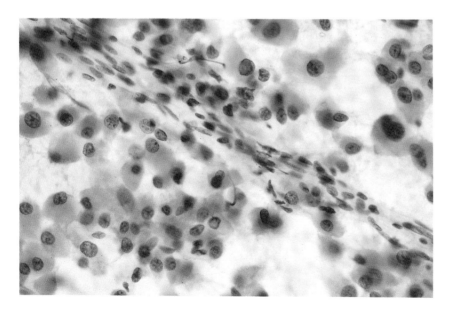

FIGURE 6–15 Well-differentiated hepato-cellular carcinoma. Dishesive sheet and single hepatocytes transgressed by proliferating endothelium. The cells have a deceptively low nuclear to cytoplasmic ratio and are punctuated by occasional larger atypical cells imitating a reactive process. The presence of transgressing endothelium is a helpful clue to the diagnosis of hepatocellular carcinoma. (Hematoxylin & eosin, ×160.)

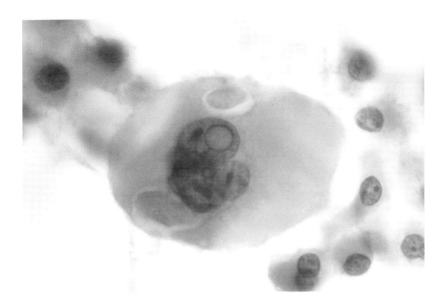

FIGURE 6–16 Well-differentiated hepatocellular carcinoma. Large malignant multinucleated hepatocyte with a low nuclear to cytoplasmic ratio similar to a dysplastic hepatocyte. The presence of an intranuclear inclusion and intracytoplasmic inclusions surrounded by characteristic halos are clues to its malignant nature. (Hematoxylin & eosin, ×250.)

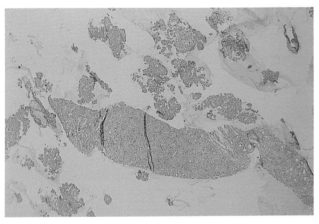

FIGURE 6–17 Well-differentiated hepatocellular carcinoma. Cell block preparation demonstrating a cirrhotic nodule surrounded by friable dishesive fragments of hepatocytes forming acini surrounded by endothelial cells, diagnostic of hepatocellular carcinoma. (Hematoxylin & eosin, ×160.)

Figures 6–15 through 6–18 illustrate another example of WDHCC in which the tumor cells form dishesive sheets transgressed by proliferating endothelial cells (Figure 6–15) punctuated with occasional multinucleated tumor cells with prominent nucleoli, intranuclear pseudo-inclusions, and eosinophilic cytoplasmic inclusions surrounded by a clear halo (Figure 6–16). These characteristic tumor cell cytoplasmic inclusions have been shown to stain positively for alpha-1-antitrypsin (AAT), AFP, and fibrinogen.[3] These cells should not be confused with dysplastic hepatocytes. The supplemental cell block in this case supported the diagnosis of WDHCC that was arising in the background of cirrhosis (Figures 6–17 and 6–18).

FIGURE 6–18 Well-differentiated hepatocellular carcinoma. Cell block preparation. High-power view of Figure 6–17 better illustrating the thickened trabeculae with acinar formation and rounded nests of hepatocytes enveloped by endothelium, architectural abnormalities diagnostic of hepatocellular carcinoma. (Hematoxylin & eosin, ×160.)

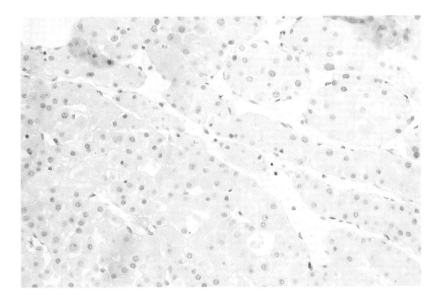

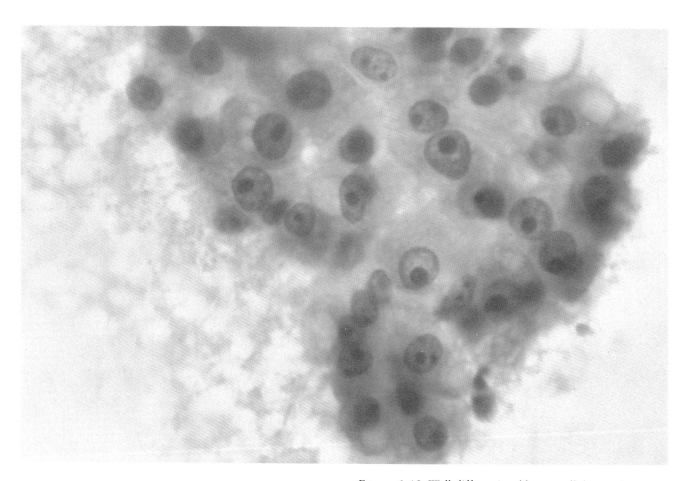

Figure 6–19 Well-differentiated hepatocellular carcinoma. Cohesive nest of atypical hepatocytes with macronucleoli not surrounded by endothelium, but with acinar formation apparent. (Papanicolaou, ×250.) (Reproduced with permission of the American Society of Clinical Pathologists. ASCP 1993 Resident In-Service Examination, slide 31.)

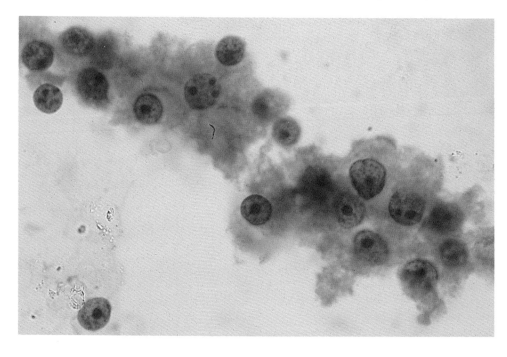

Figure 6–20 Well-differentiated hepatocellular carcinoma. Irregular cluster of hepatocytes with slightly increased nuclear to cytoplasmic ratio, prominent nucleoli, and only subtle nuclear crowding, features that could be confused with a reactive process. (Hematoxylin & eosin, ×250.)

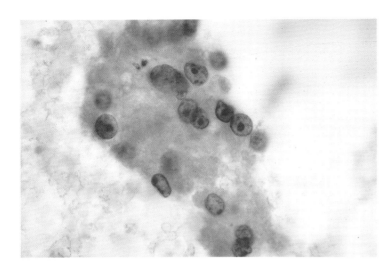

FIGURE 6–21 Well-differentiated hepatocellular carcinoma. Small cluster of slightly atypical hepatocytes forming an acinus. (Hematoxylin & eosin, ×250.)

Well-differentiated hepatocellular carcinoma is most difficult to diagnose when the smear architecture does not illustrate rounded nests or thick trabeculae and neither peripheral nor transgressing endothelium is present. In these cases, individual cell group cytomorphology must be closely examined. In some cases, large cohesive groups with only focal acinar formation and macronucleoli will be apparent (Figure 6–19); in others, the atypia may be more subtle with slight hyperchromasia, prominent nucleoli, and nuclear envelope irregularities (Figure 6–20), or small groups of hepatocytes forming an acinus (Figures 6–21 and 6–22) may be appreciated. Cell block preparations, no matter how scant the tissue fragments, are almost always helpful in these cases (Figure 6–23).

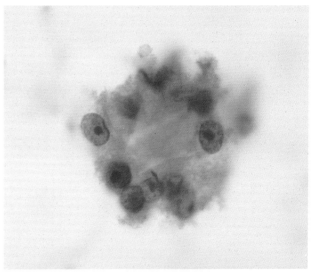

FIGURE 6–22 Well-differentiated hepatocellular carcinoma. Slightly atypical hepatocytes forming an acinus. (Hematoxylin & eosin, ×250.)

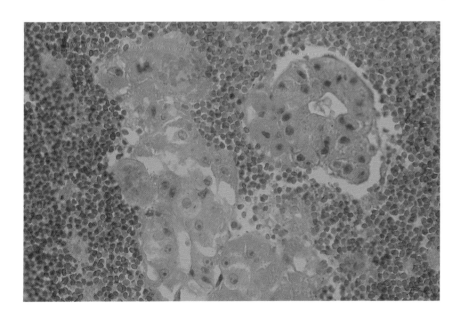

FIGURE 6–23 Well-differentiated hepatocellular carcinoma. Cell block preparation showing tiny fragments of well-differentiated hepatocellular carcinoma with atypical acinar architecture. (Hematoxylin & eosin, ×80.)

The primary differential diagnosis with WDHCC is a benign reactive or neoplastic process such as cirrhosis, liver cell adenoma, or focal nodular hyperplasia (FNH) (see Chapter 5). Metastatic malignancies that often closely mimic WDHCC include granular renal cell carcinoma and malignant melanoma. Renal cell carcinoma (Figure 6–24) with its round central nucleus, macronucleolus, and abundant granular cytoplasm closely resembles hepatocytes. Subtle differences include a tendency to cluster in irregular groups often with a fibrovascular core rather than in rounded nests and trabeculae with peripheral or transgressing endothelium. The macronucleoli in renal cell carcinoma also tend to be bigger and surrounded by a distinct clear zone ("owl's eye" nucleus). Some HCCs may also have similar appearing nuclei, so in some cases you may have to resort to clinical evaluation to absolutely rule out a renal metastasis. Malignant melanoma can mimic the dishesive cells of WDHCC (Figures 6–25 and 6–26). Despite the similar-appearing rounded nuclei with prominent nucleoli and often intranuclear inclusions, the nuclei are more often eccentric and much more pleomorphic, and the N/C ratio tends to be uniformly more elevated than in WDHCC. In some cases, only special studies such as immunocytochemistry will definitively differentiate the two.

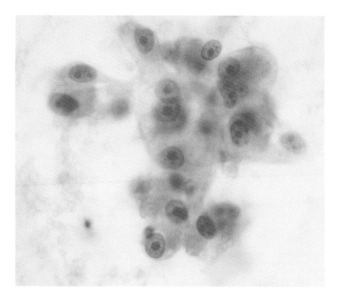

FIGURE 6–24 Renal cell carcinoma, granular cell type. Subtle differences from hepatocellular carcinoma include a tendency to form irregular groups, often with a fibrovascular core, and macronucleoli with a clear zone giving an "owl's eye" appearance.

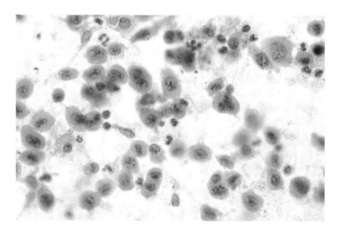

FIGURE 6–25 Malignant melanoma, epithelial cell type. This type of melanoma with its round polygonal single cell population, round nuclei, and sometimes small, inconspicuous nucleoli and dense cytoplasm resembles hepatocellular carcinoma. (Papanicolaou, ×160.)

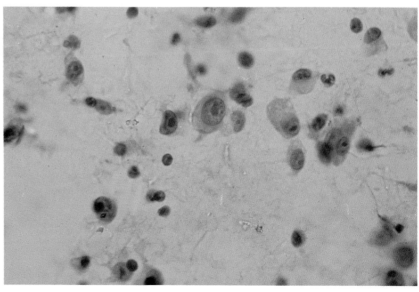

FIGURE 6–26 Malignant melanoma, epithelial cell type. Melanoma cells are distinguished by their more uniformly increased nuclear to cytoplasmic ratio, eccentric nuclei, and greater degree of pleomorphism. (Hematoxylin & eosin, ×160.)

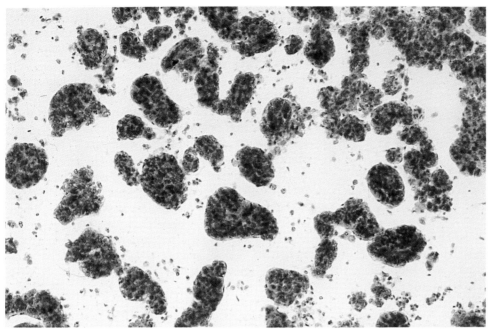

FIGURE 6–27 Moderately differentiated hepatocellular carcinoma. Typical smear pattern with rounded nests and trabeculae surrounded by endothelium (Papanicolaou, ×160.)

Moderately Differentiated

Moderately differentiated hepatocellular carcinoma (MDHCC) is the least difficult to diagnose on smears because not only do the cells have obviously malignant characteristics, there is usually relatively good preservation of hepatocytic features. The aspirate smear pattern is often typical of HCC in general, with numerous cohesive nests and thick trabeculae (Figure 6–27) that can sometimes be quite long and twisted (Figure 6–28). Preservation of hepatocytic features with round, central nuclei, prominent nucleoli, and relatively abundant granular cytoplasm is often appreciated (Figure 6–29).

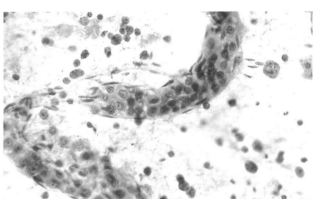

FIGURE 6–28 Moderately differentiated hepatocellular carcinoma. Long, twisted, thickened trabeculum lined by endothelium. Preservation of hepatocytic features is present with polygonal cell shape and round central nuclei. (Papanicolaou, ×100.)

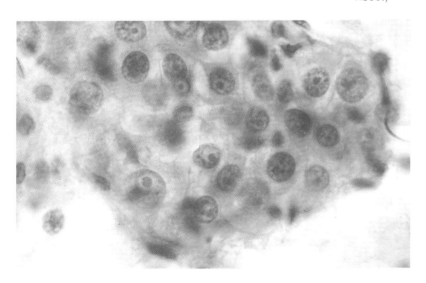

FIGURE 6–29 Moderately differentiated hepatocellular carcinoma. Cohesive nests surrounded by endothelium with preservation of hepatocytic features represented by polygonal shape, round central nuclei, prominent nucleoli (which may sometimes have an "owl's eye" appearance like renal cell carcinoma), and abundant granular cytoplasm. (Papanicolaou, ×250.)

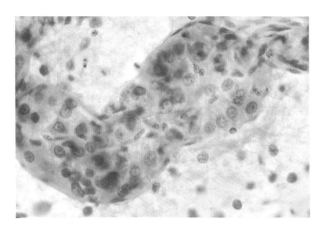

FIGURE 6–30 Moderately differentiated hepatocellular carcinoma. Malignant hepatocytes with preservation of hepatocytic features forming a twisted trabeculum enveloped by endothelium. (Papanicolaou, ×100.)

The presence of endothelium is the most helpful feature in our experience[7]; it may be peripheral around groups with well-preserved hepatocytic features (Figure 6–30) or not so well-preserved features (Figure 6–31), or present transgressing loosely cohesive sheets (Figures 6–32 and 6–33). We have not seen these patterns of endothelial proliferation in a series of 100 metastatic tumors we reviewed that included adenocarcinoma, melanoma, squamous cell carcinoma, and lymphoma.[7] The presence of intranuclear pseudo-inclusions and acinar formation are also more commonly associated with MDHCC than WDHCC (Figure 6–34). The presence of numerous atypical naked nuclei is a feature often associated with high-grade HCC and has been reported as a very helpful feature in suggesting a hepatic origin to an obviously malignant tumor[8] (Figure 6–35). These naked nuclei may be single or clustered (Figure 6–36).

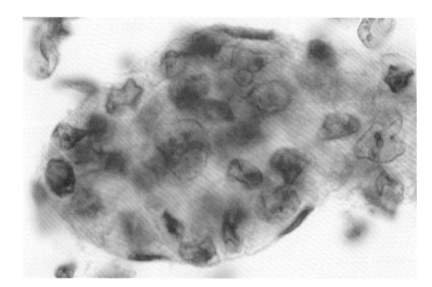

FIGURE 6–31 Moderately differentiated hepatocellular carcinoma. Malignant cells with not so well-preserved hepatocytic features surrounded by endothelium, a clue to their origin. (Papanicolaou, ×250.)

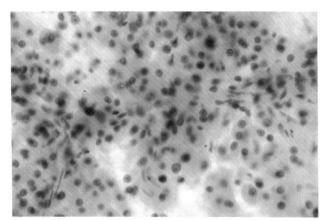

FIGURE 6–32 Moderately differentiated hepatocellular carcinoma. Dishesive pleomorphic hepatocytes centrally transgressed by proliferating endothelium (Papanicolaou, ×100.)

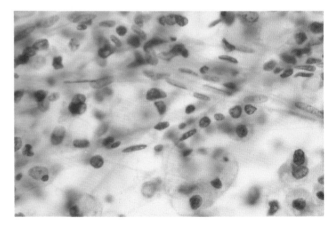

FIGURE 6–33 Moderately differentiated hepatocellular carcinoma. High magnification view of the same tumor in Figure 6–32 demonstrating the centrally transgressing endothelium among dishesive malignant hepatocytes. (Papanicolaou, ×250.)

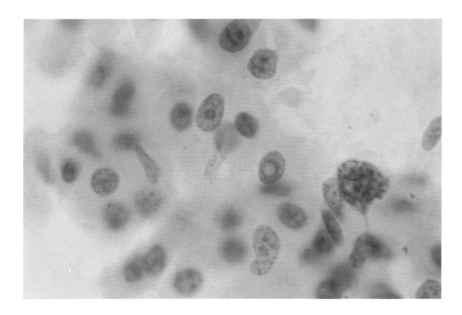

FIGURE 6–34 Moderately differentiated hepatocellular carcinoma. Acinar formation and intranuclear inclusions are common in moderately differentiated tumors. (Papanicolaou, ×250.)

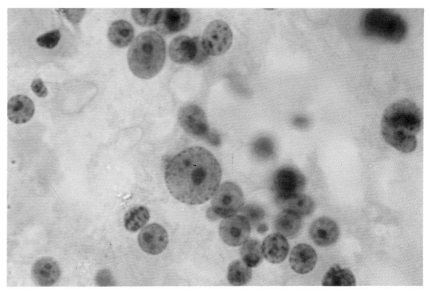

FIGURE 6–35 Moderately differentiated hepatocellular carcinoma. Scattered naked tumor nuclei are a helpful feature in discerning hepatic origin. (Papanicolaou, ×250.)

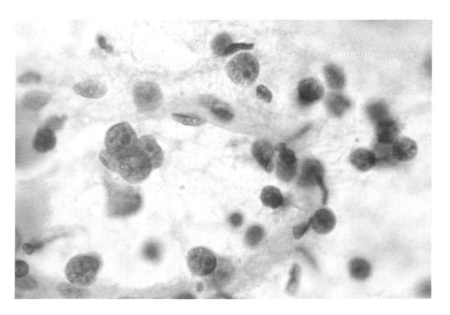

FIGURE 6–36 Moderately differentiated hepatocellular carcinoma. Naked hepatocytic nuclei may occur singly or in clusters. (Papanicolaou, ×250.)

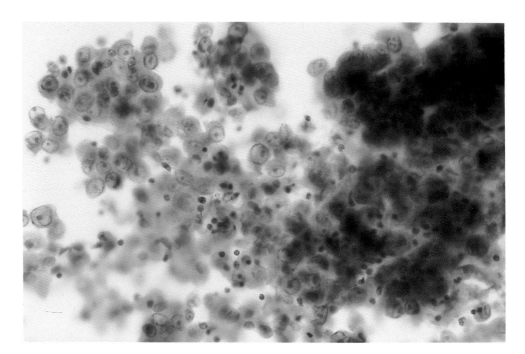

FIGURE 6–37 Poorly differentiated hepatocellular carcinoma. Dishesive irregular cluster of malignant cells with poorly preserved hepatocytic features. (Papanicolaou, ×100.)

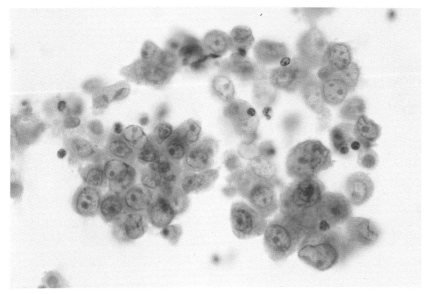

FIGURE 6–38 Poorly differentiated hepatocellular carcinoma. Poor preservation of hepatocytic features with extremely high nuclear to cytoplasmic ratio and prominent nucleoli. Scant granular cytoplasm is apparent with some cells. (Papanicolaou, ×160.)

Poorly Differentiated

Poorly differentiated hepatocellular carcinoma (PDHCC) is not difficult to interpret as malignant but is almost always difficult to interpret as hepatocytic in origin on routine aspirate smear preparations. Smears are frequently very cellular, composed of irregular aggregates of loosely cohesive cells (Figure 6–37) with a high N/C ratio and little to no preservation of hepatocytic features (Figure 6–38). Some groups may simulate a thick trabeculum (Figure 6–39), and the presence of endothelial cells may be very focal and difficult to find but, when present in either the peripheral or transgressing pattern, indicates hepatic origin[7] (Figure 6–40). Other features suggestive of hepatocytic origin include a graduated spectrum of atypia in the same cluster, from poorly differentiated malignant hepatocytes to benign reactive hepatocytes (Figure 6–41); the association of tumor with cirrhosis (Figure 6–42) or hemochromatosis (Figure 6–43); the presence of naked tumor nuclei (Figure 6–44); and the presence of multinucleated tumor giant cells (Figure 6–45). Tumor necrosis and mitoses may also be present. Only the production of bile by the tumor cells is pathognomonic of hepatic origin (Figure 6–46).

Cell block preparations are important for providing tissue easily accessible for special studies but also often demonstrate tissue fragments with better preserved hepatocytic features (Figure 6–47) and architectural changes diagnostic of HCC (Figure 6–48).

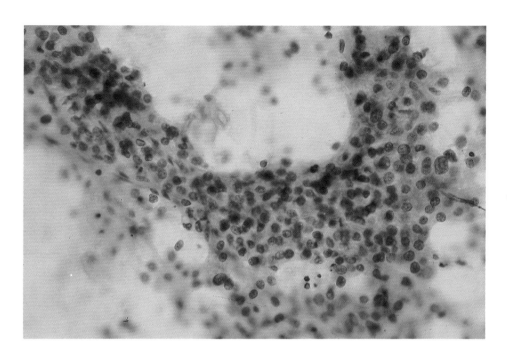

FIGURE 6–39 Poorly differentiated hepatocellular carcinoma. A long, irregular cluster of malignant hepatocytes simulating a trabeculum without obvious peripheral endothelium. (Papanicolaou, ×100.)

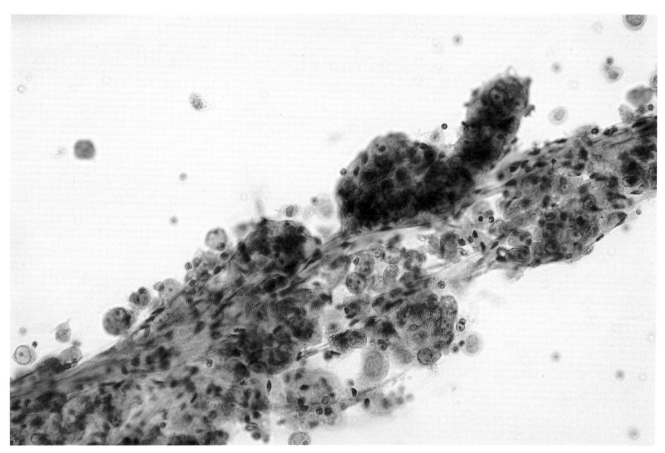

FIGURE 6–40 Poorly differentiated hepatocellular carcinoma. The presence of peripheral and transgressing endothelium is indicative of hepatic origin. (Papanicolaou, ×100.)

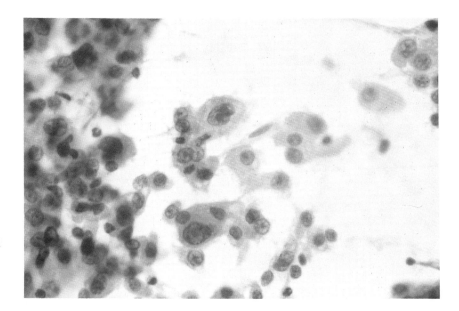

FIGURE 6–41 Poorly differentiated hepatocellular carcinoma. A graduated spectrum of atypia from poorly differentiated malignant hepatocytes to benign hepatocytes is a feature suggestive of hepatic origin. (Papanicolaou, ×250.)

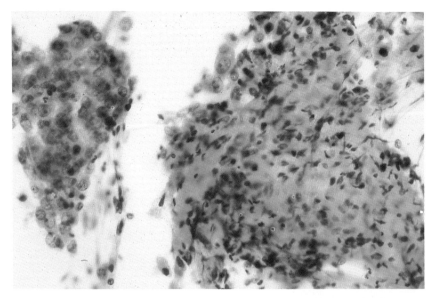

FIGURE 6–42 Poorly differentiated hepatocellular carcinoma. The presence of a background of cirrhosis is helpful in suggesting a hepatic origin of the tumor. (Papanicolaou, ×160.)

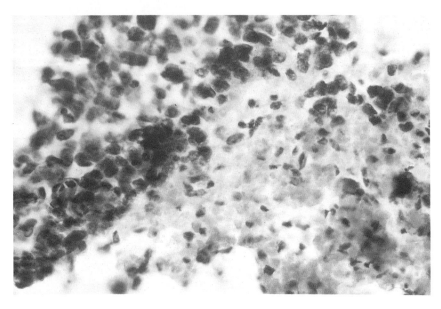

FIGURE 6–43 Poorly differentiated hepatocellular carcinoma. The association with hemachromatosis is a feature suggestive of hepatic origin of the tumor. (Hematoxylin & eosin, ×100.)

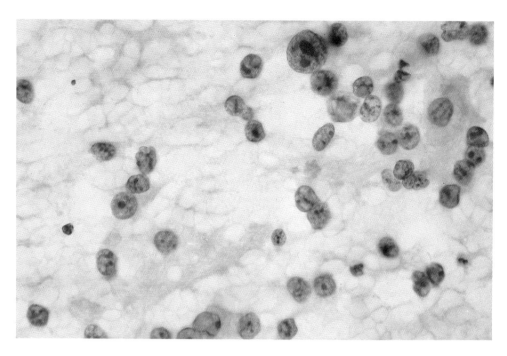

FIGURE 6–44 Poorly differentiated hepatocellular carcinoma. The presence of naked tumor nuclei resembling those in clusters is suggestive of hepatic origin. (Papanicolaou, ×160.)

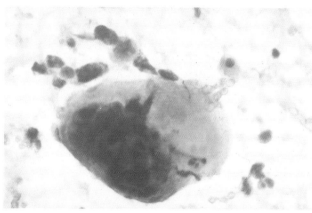

FIGURE 6–45 Poorly differentiated hepatocellular carcinoma. The presence of multinucleated tumor giant cells is common and suggestive of hepatic origin. (Hematoxylin & eosin, ×160.)

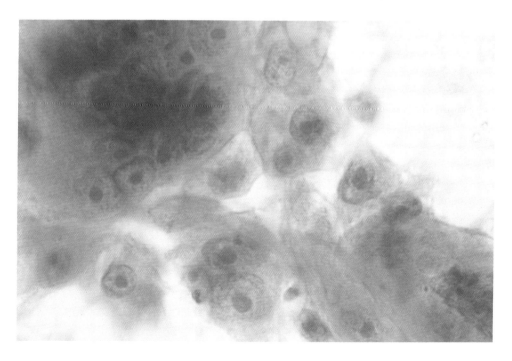

FIGURE 6–46 Poorly differentiated hepatocellular carcinoma. The identification of bile is the only pathognomonic feature of hepatic origin. (Papanicolaou, ×250.)

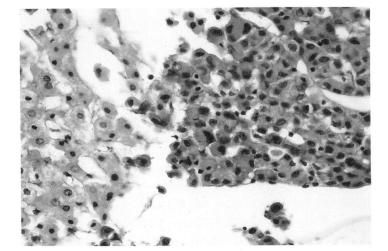

FIGURE 6–47 Poorly differentiated hepatocellular carcinoma. Cell block preparations often demonstrate better preserved cytologic and architectural features diagnostic of hepatocellular carcinoma. (Hematoxylin & eosin, ×100.)

FIGURE 6–48 Poorly differentiated hepatocellular carcinoma. Higher magnification view of Figure 6–47 showing acinar formation, endothelial wrapping, and focally relatively well-preserved hepatocytic features. (Hematoxylin & eosin, ×160.)

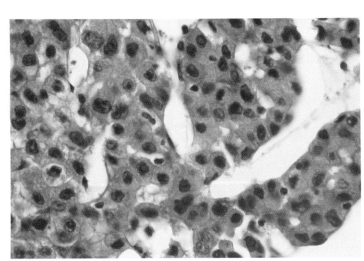

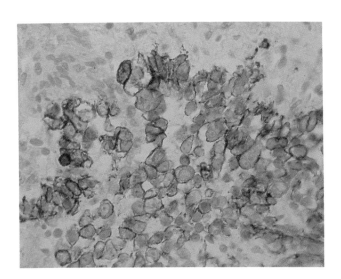

FIGURE 6–49 Poorly differentiated hepatocellular carcinoma. Cells stain positively for alpha-fetoprotein. (Immunoperoxidase, ×100.)

The best immunocytochemical profile used for tumors suspected of being HCC includes AFP, keratins CAM 5.2 and AE1 (or AE1,3), and carcinoembryonic antigen (CEA). Positive staining with AFP is the most helpful and may be detected in tumor cells with or without elevated serum levels.[3] HCC is generally positive for AFP (Figure 6–49) but may be negative. Other tumors that stain positively for AFP include endodermal sinus tumor, embryonal carcinoma, and carcinoma of the lung and stomach. One study[9] has shown that in most cases keratin CAM 5.2 will stain hepatocytes—benign (Figure 6–50A) or malignant (Figure 6–50B)—in addition to cholangiocarcinoma and metastatic adenocarcinoma, whereas keratin AE1 (or AE1,3 in our experience) fails to stain hepatocytes of HCC (Figure 6–50C) or benign liver, while positively staining cholangiocarcinoma and metastatic adenocarcinoma (Figure 6–50D). Carcinoembryonic antigen, although typically positive in adenocarcinomas, has a cannilicular or apical staining pattern in HCC[9,10] (Figure 6–51). AAT, although generally considered nonspecific,[9] is often positive in HCC.

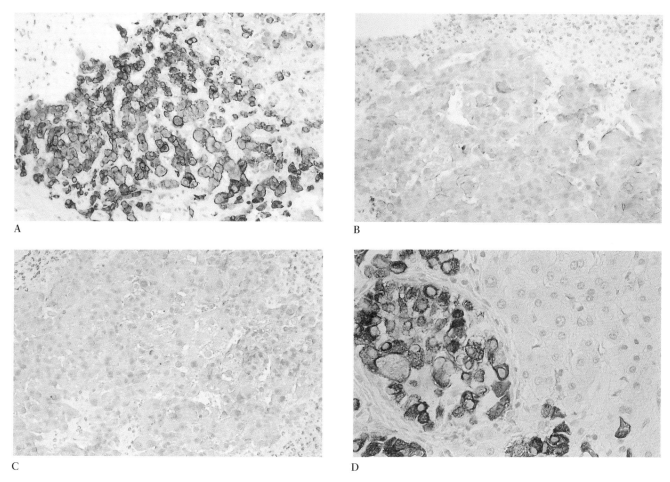

A

B

C

D

FIGURE 6–50 A. Keratin CAM 5.2 stains the cells of normal liver. B. Hepatocytes of hepatocellular caracinoma also stain with keratin CAM 5.2, in this case faintly. C. Keratin AE1,3 fails to stain hepatocytes of most hepatocellular carcino-mas. D. This metastatic adenocarcinoma stains positively for keratin AE1,3, but the adjacent benign hepatocytes do not. (A through D, Immunoperoxidase, ×100.)

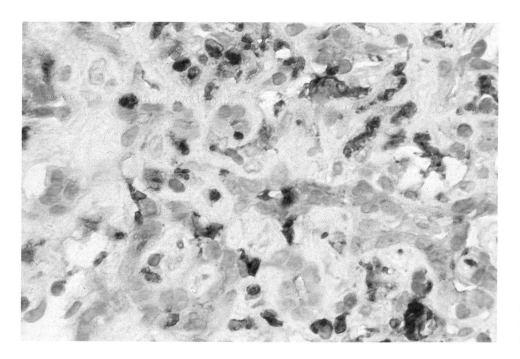

FIGURE 6–51 Poorly differentiated hepatocellular carcinoma. Carcinoembryonic antigen has an apical and cannilicular staining pattern. (Immunoperoxidase, ×160.)

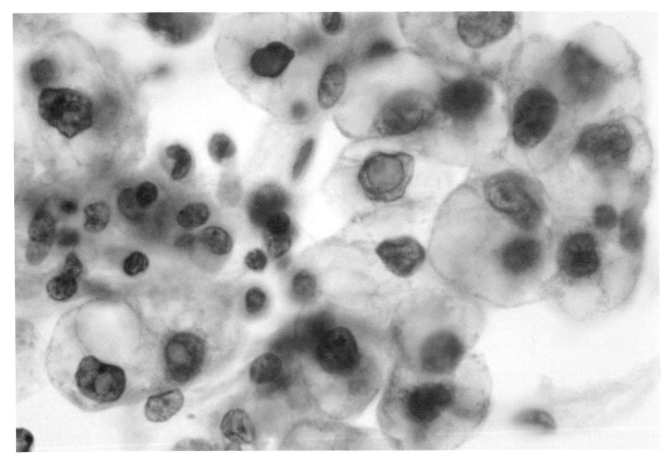

FIGURE 6–52 Clear cell hepatocellular carcinoma. Hepatocytes have vacuolated clear cytoplasm resulting from glycogen and fat. (Papanicolaou, ×250.)

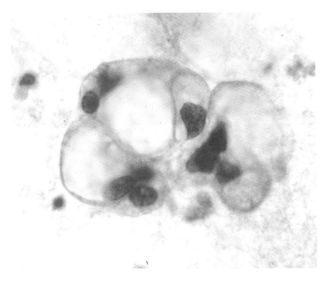

FIGURE 6–53 Clear cell hepatocellular carcinoma. Vacuoles may be small and multiple or large and single, sometimes resembling signet ring cells. (Papanicolaou, ×250.)

Variants

Clear Cell

Clear cell HCC is a well-established variant[4,5,11,12] that must be differentiated from metastatic clear cell tumors of the kidney, adrenal gland, and ovary. Tumors are composed of a clear cell population that varies from 30 to 100 percent[4,12] the clear cytoplasmic features resulting from glycogen and fat (Figure 6–52). The cytoplasmic vacuoles vary from small and multiple to large and single and may mimic signet ring cells (Figure 6–53). There is generally a non–clear cell HCC component as well, which aids in the identification of a hepatic origin[4,5,12] (Figure 6–54). Endothelium is a very helpful feature that is often present either peripherally or as penetrating or transgressing bands running through loosely cohesive sheets of hepatocytes (Figures 6–54 and 6–55) typical of that described for non–clear cell HCC. The cell block preparations in this case (Figure 6–56) provided tissue for immunocytochemistry, but morphologically were less diagnostic than the aspirate smears.

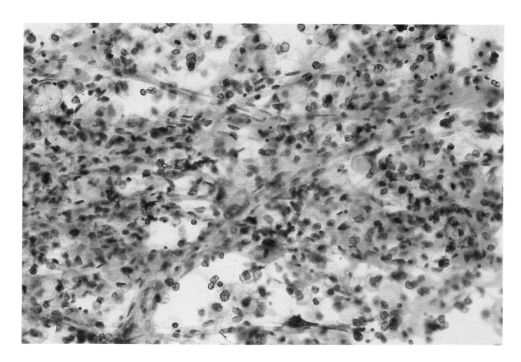

FIGURE 6–54 Clear cell hepatocellular carcinoma. The presence of transgressing endothelium and a non–clear cell component are helpful features in determining hepatic origin. (Papanicolaou, ×80).

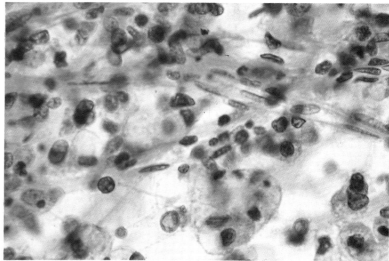

FIGURE 6–55 Clear cell hepatocellular carcinoma. Higher magnification view of Figure 6–54 better illustrating the transgressing endothelium. (Papanicolaou, ×250.)

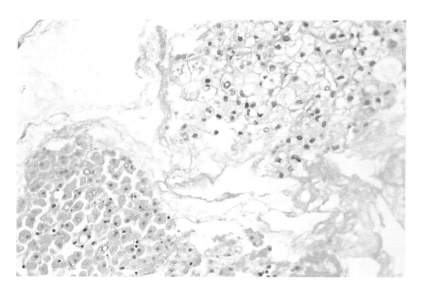

FIGURE 6–56 Clear cell hepatocellular carcinoma. Cell block preparation showing fragment of bland appearing clear cell tumor adjacent to normal hepatocytes. (Hematoxylin & eosin, ×40.)

The differential diagnosis primarily includes metastatic clear cell tumors of the adrenal gland, ovary, and kidney. Probably the most difficult differential diagnosis is with metastatic renal cell carcinoma, clear cell type (Figure 6–57). The distinguishing features are the same as discussed for the granular renal cell carcinoma, namely, renal tumors have a tendency to cluster in small irregular groups not associated with visible endothelium and have a characteristic "owl's eye" macronucleolus surrounded by a clear zone. These differences may be very subtle, and often a renal tumor is excluded solely by the lack of clinical history.

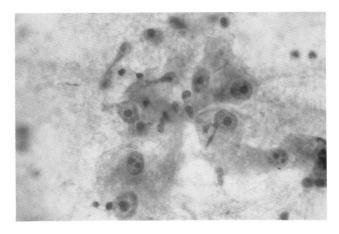

FIGURE 6–57 Renal cell carcinoma, clear cell type. The tendency to form in small clusters usually associated with vessels, the lack of peripheral and/or transgressing endothelium, and a slightly more pronounced macronucleolus often with a halo are features more in keeping with this tumor than hepatocellular carcinoma. (Papanicolaou, ×250.)

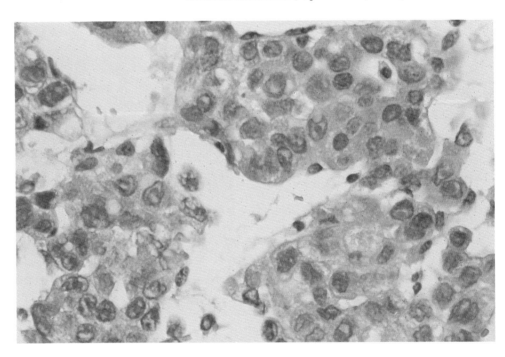

FIGURE 6–58 Acinar cell variant hepatocellular carcinoma. Acinar formation is apparent in endothelial wrapped nests of malignant hepatocytes with relatively well-preserved hepatocytic features. (Hematoxylin & eosin, ×160.)

Acinar Cell

Acinar cell HCC presents as a typical MDHCC on smears. Smears are cellular, often with endothelially wrapped cohesive nests and trabeculae composed of obviously malignant cells but with relatively well-preserved hepatocytic features. The cells have pleomorphic nuclei with irregular nuclear membranes, intranuclear pseudoinclusions, and frequent prominent nucleoli. Acini may be apparent in many cell clusters (Figure 6–58). The presence of acini is a common and helpful diagnostic feature of many HCCs of all levels of differentiation, but when they are a predominant feature as usually evi-

denced on cell block preparations only (Figure 6–59), the acinar variant label is appropriate. The presence of apparent "gland formation" on cell block preparations introduces adenocarcinoma (primary or metastatic) into the differential diagnosis. On close inspection of the cells, however, it is apparent that the "glands" are not true glands because they lack a basement membrane, and that they are also composed of the same cells that form sheets between the "glands" (Figure 6–60). A mucicarmine stain will be negative (Figure 6–61). These features along with the more typical HCC appearance on smears should lead to the correct diagnosis.

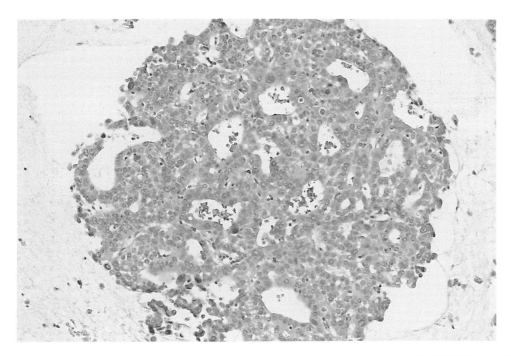

FIGURE 6–59 Acinar cell variant hepatocellular carcinoma. Cell block preparation shows confluent "gland" formation introducing adenocarcinoma into the differential diagnosis. (Hematoxylin & eosin, ×40.)

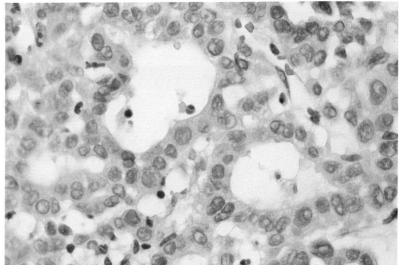

FIGURE 6–60 Acinar cell variant hepatocellular carcinoma. The "glands" are not true glands for lack of a basement membrane. The cells between the glands are also the same as those composing the glands. (Papanicolaou, ×160.)

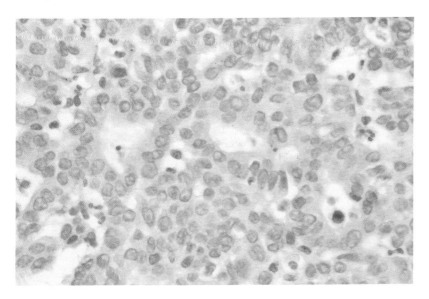

FIGURE 6–61 Acinar cell variant hepatocellular carcinoma. Special stain for mucin is negative. (Mucicarmine, ×160.)

Fibrolamellar

Fibrolamellar HCC distinguishes itself from other forms of HCC in both its biologic and morphologic characteristics. It is predominately a tumor of young adults, with a 14 to 54 percent incidence in patients under 35 years of age in almost a 1:1 male to female ratio.[13-16] Typical HCC occurs in older (average age 52 years) men, most commonly in a cirrhotic liver. Seventy-five percent of fibrolamellar HCCs, however, arise in the noncirrhotic liver, and over half the patients have tumor confined to the liver at the time of diagnosis.[13-16] In addition, whereas HCC is commonly associated with significantly elevated serum AFP levels, patients with fibrolamellar HCC seldom have elevated levels.[14,16] Some patients may have an elevated serum unsaturated vitamin B_{12} binding capacity, a feature unique to this type of HCC.[17]

Grossly, fibrolamellar tumors most often present as a single mass and may resemble FNH (Figure 6–62). Microscopically, fibrolamellar HCC is unique and distinct from FNH, sclerosing HCC, and sclerosing metastases by the presence of thick, parallel bundles of acellular collagen that separate bands of malignant eosinophilic (oxyphilic) hepatocytes (Figure 6–63). The presence of this prominent fibrotic component often results in a paucicellular aspirate. The classic cytomorphologic picture is composed of numerous dishesive oxyphilic hepatocytes with frankly malignant pleomorphic, hyperchromatic nuclei, macronucleoli, and abundant granular cytoplasm (Figure 6–64). More often, however, the smear will be paucicellular, composed of isolated oxyphilic cells and/or naked nuclei that frequently demonstrate characteristic cytoplasmic hyaline inclusion bodies and intranuclear pseudo-inclusions (Figure 6–65). Fibroblasts and lymphocytes may occasionally be present (Figure 6–66). The diagnosis of HCC—much less fibrolamellar HCC—may be difficult on such paucicellular smears. Intranuclear cytoplasmic hyaline inclusions are also characteristic of reactive hepatocytes in alcoholic cirrhosis. The commonly encountered pale bodies described on histopathologic sections are difficult if not impossible to appreciate on such paucicellular smears. Cell block preparations of tissue fragments (Figures 6–67 and 6–68) may be necessary to make a definitive diagnosis.

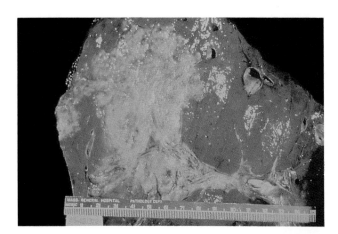

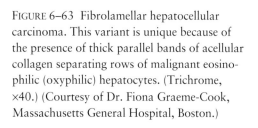

FIGURE 6–63 Fibrolamellar hepatocellular carcinoma. This variant is unique because of the presence of thick parallel bands of acellular collagen separating rows of malignant eosinophilic (oxyphilic) hepatocytes. (Trichrome, ×40.) (Courtesy of Dr. Fiona Graeme-Cook, Massachusetts General Hospital, Boston.)

FIGURE 6–62 Fibrolamellar hepatocellular carcinoma. Gross tumor may resemble focal nodular hyperplasia. (Courtesy of Dr. Fiona Graeme-Cook, Massachusetts General Hospital, Boston.)

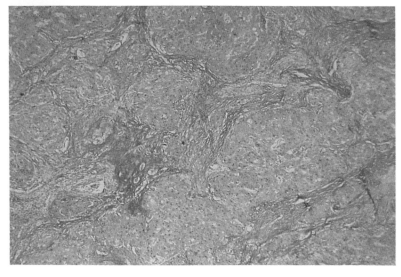

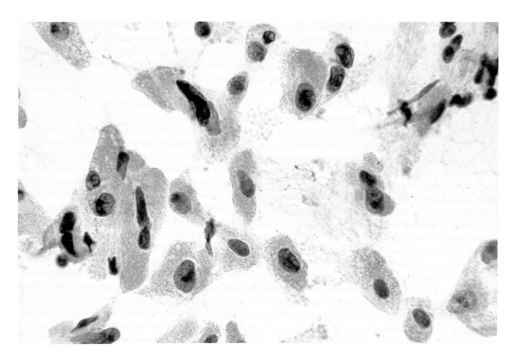

FIGURE 6–64 Fibrolamellar hepatocellular carcinoma. The classic smear is composed of dishesive oxyphilic hepatocytes with pleomorphic, hyperchromatic nuclei, macronucleoli, and abundant granular cytoplasm. (Papanicolaou, ×160.)

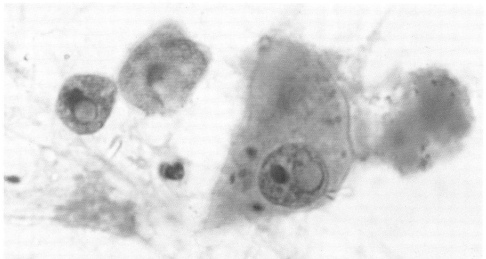

FIGURE 6–65 Fibrolamellar hepatocellular carcinoma. Paucicellular smear composed of atypical hepatocytes with macronucleoli, intranuclear inclusions, and characteristic cytoplasmic hyalin inclusion bodies. (Papanicolaou, ×250.)

FIGURE 6–66 Fibrolamellar hepatocellular carcinoma. Oxyphilic hepatocytes may be associated with fibroblasts and lymphocytes demonstrating smear artifact. (Hematoxylin & eosin, ×100.)

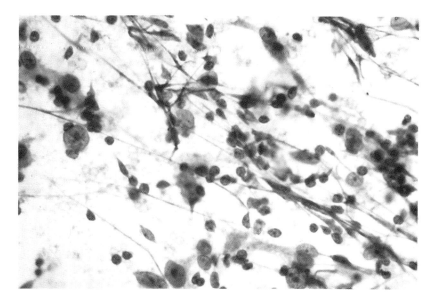

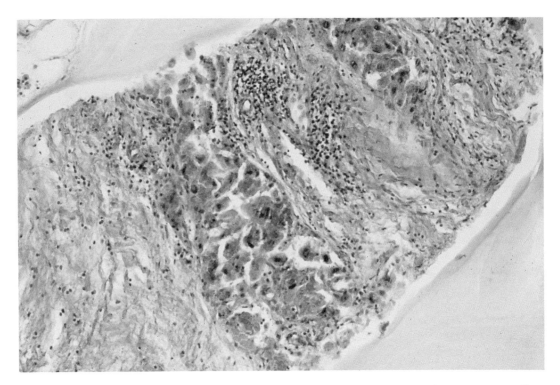

FIGURE 6–67 Fibrolamellar hepatocellular carcinoma. Cell block preparation beautifully demonstrates the thick parallel bands of collagen separating malignant oxyphilic hepatocytes.

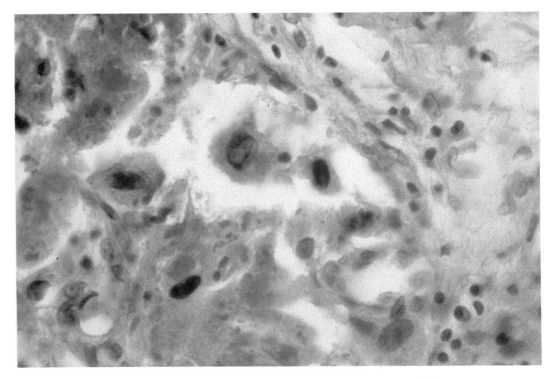

FIGURE 6–68 Fibrolamellar hepatocellular carcinoma. Higher magnification view of malignant hepatocytes in Figure 6–67 illustrating intranuclear inclusions and characteristic cytoplasmic hyalin inclusions. (Hematoxylin & eosin, ×250.)

HEPATOBLASTOMA

Hepatoblastoma (HB) represents the most common malignant primary hepatic tumor in young children.[18] Histologically, this tumor is classified as epithelial (with fetal and embryonal subtypes), mixed epithelial and mesenchymal, and anaplastic or small-cell undifferentiated.[20–21] The fetal-epithelial type has the best prognosis [21,22] and the small-cell undifferentiated the worst,[19,22,23] with surgical resection the only chance for cure in any type.[19,21,24]

The epithelial type is the more common and widely reported example in the cytology literature.[25–28] The fetal embryonal subtypes may be very difficult to distinguish from one another on smears alone[28] and contain cytomorphologic features that overlap with those of HCC.[26] Smears are very cellular and contain mostly cohesive nests, flat sheets, and thick cords or trabeculae of small, round-to-oval, crowded, atypical hepatocytes (Figures 6–69 and 6–70). Cells have a high N/C ratio with round to slightly eccentric nuclei with overlapping, hyperchromasia and nucleoli, and vacuolated to granular cytoplasm (Figures 6–71 and 6–72).

Acinar formation and naked tumor nuclei are common.[26,28] The presence of peripheral or transgressing endothelium on smear preparations has not been described. Extramedullary hematopoiesis and/or extracellular matrix material (osteoid) may also be present in HB but not in HCC[26] and thus are helpful distinguishing findings.

The mixed epithelial and mesenchymal type HB contains a spindle cell or mesenchymal component in addition to an epithelial component similar to that in the epithelial type but with more pleomorphism of cell size, shape, and nuclear features.[26]

The small-cell undifferentiated type HB is cytomorphologically similar to other small round-cell tumors of childhood and depends on immunocytochemistry and electron microscopy for definitive diagnosis.[29]

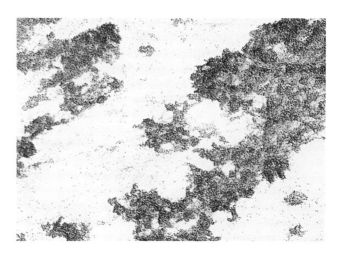

FIGURE 6–69 Hepatoblastoma. Irregular flat sheets of atypical hepatocytes. (Papanicolaou, ×40.)

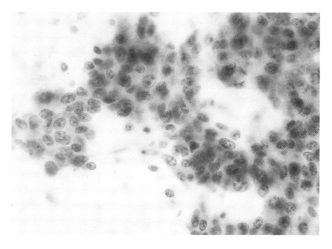

FIGURE 6–70 Hepatoblastoma. The neoplastic hepatocytes have a uniformly increased nuclear to cytoplasmic ratio, round nuclei, small nucleoli, and moderate amounts of vacuolated to granular cytoplasm. (Papanicolaou, ×160.)

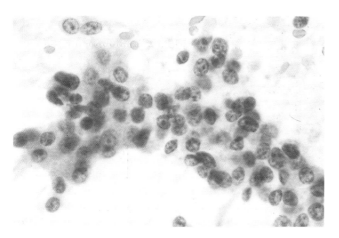

FIGURE 6–71 Hepatoblastoma. Irregular trabeculum of atypical hepatocytes without endothelial wrapping. (Papanicolaou, ×160.)

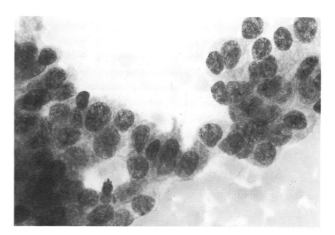

FIGURE 6–72 Hepatoblastoma. Atypical hepatocytes with high nuclear to cytoplasmic ratio and moderate amounts of granular cytoplasm. (May-Grünwald-Giemsa, ×250.)

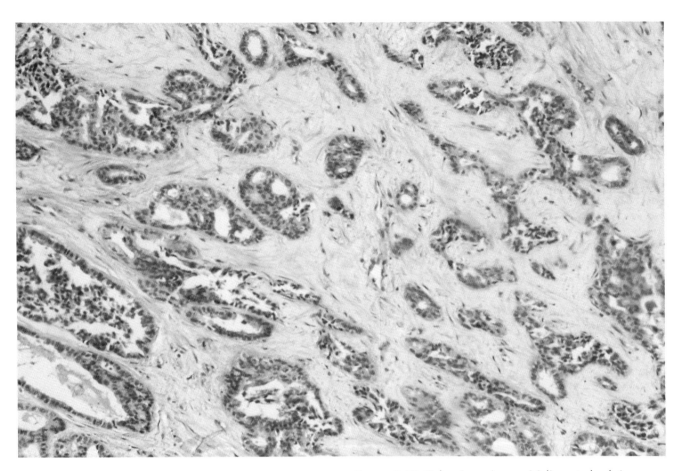

FIGURE 6–73 Colangiocarcinoma. Malignant glands in a dense fibrotic stroma are a characteristic feature. (Hematoxylin & eosin, ×40.)

CHOLANGIOCARCINOMA

Cholangiocarcinoma (CC) is a relatively rare neoplasm of the bile duct system occurring much less commonly in the liver than HCC.[30] Like the typical HCC, it is a tumor of older men, but unlike the typical HCC, it does not commonly occur in the cirrhotic liver.[30] It is associated with primary sclerosing cholangitis,[30] ulcerative colitis,[31] Clonorchis sinensis parasitic infestation,[32] and exposure to chemical toxins such as thorotrast.[33,34]

Histologically, CC is an adenocarcinoma composed of cuboidal to columnar cells with clear to eosinophilic cytoplasm in a dense fibrotic stroma (Figure 6–73). Mucin is generally detectable and occasionally abundant, a characteristic distinguishing it from HCC.

Aspirate smears of the most common histologic type of CC demonstrate a population of cells in irregular three-dimensional clusters that often resemble groups of atypical bile duct epithelium (Figure 6–74). Rounded nests with acinar formation and cells with prominent nucleoli may resemble HCC (Figure 6–75). The nucleoli are not the large eosinophilic macronucleoli seen in some HCCs, and peripheral endothelium is absent.[7]

Glandular cribforming may be appreciated in some groups (Figure 6–76). In general, however, it is a tumor easily identifiable as an adenocarcinoma, but with nonspecific features (Figures 6–77 and 6–78). It is indistinguishable from ductal carcinoma of the pancreas and is often impossible to differentiate from other metastatic adenocarcinomas.

Cell block preparations may be very helpful in providing tissue fragments that not only demonstrate the characteristic (but nonspecific) sclerotic stroma (Figure 6–79) but may also show foci illustrating an in situ component of the tumor (Figure 6–80), a feature diagnostic of bile duct origin.

A positive mucin stain will confirm the presence of an adenocarcinoma and rule out HCC but will not differentiate CC from a metastasis. Immunoperoxidase stains may be helpful in differentiating CC from HCC, but not from metastatic adenocarcinoma.[9] Both CC and metastatic adenocarcinomas are positive for CEA and keratin CAM 5.2 and AE1 (or AE1, 3), whereas HCC is typically positive for keratin CAM 5.2 only, and CC is rarely positive for AFP and AAT.

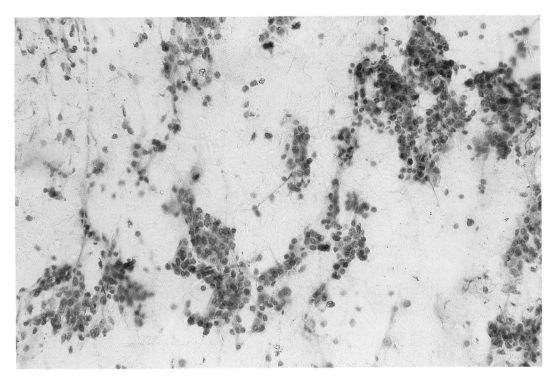

FIGURE 6–74 Colangiocarcinoma. The aspirate smears demonstrate irregular three-dimensional clusters that resemble groups of atypical bile duct epithelium in a reactive process. (Hematoxylin & eosin, ×100.)

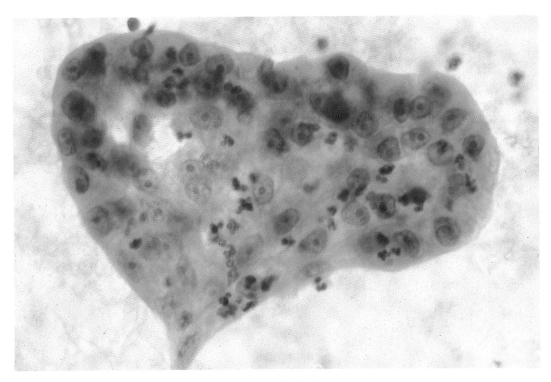

FIGURE 6–75 Colangiocarcinoma. Rounded nests with gland formation and prominent nucleoli may resemble hepatocellular carcinoma. (Papanicolaou, ×160.)

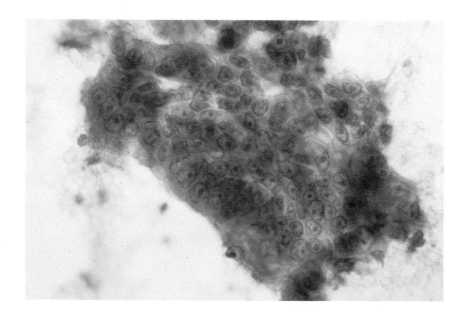

FIGURE 6–76 Colangiocarcinoma. Glandular cribriforming may be apparent in some groups. (Hematoxylin & eosin, ×160.)

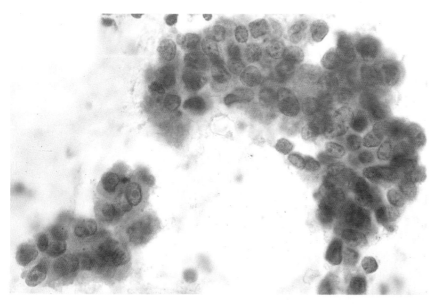

FIGURE 6–77 Colangiocarcinoma. Features of adenocarcinoma are present but nonspecific. (Hematoxylin & eosin, ×160.)

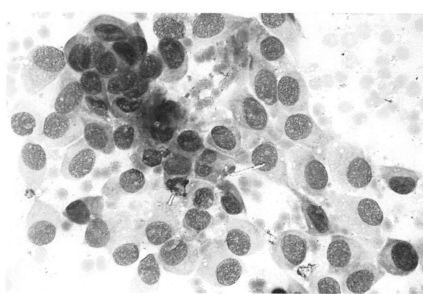

FIGURE 6–78 Colangiocarcinoma. Features of adenocarcinoma are apparent but nonspecific (May-Grünwald-Giesma, ×160.)

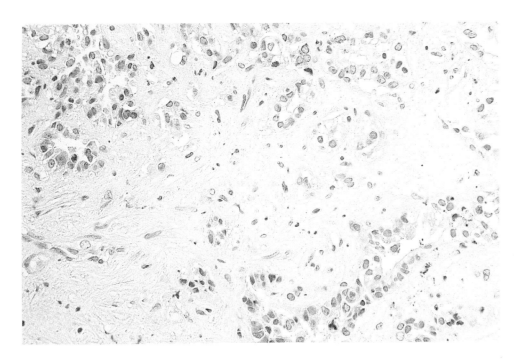

FIGURE 6–79 Colangiocar-cinoma. Cell block prepara-tion illustrating the characteristic but nonspe-cific fibrotic stroma. (Hematoxylin & eosin, ×40.)

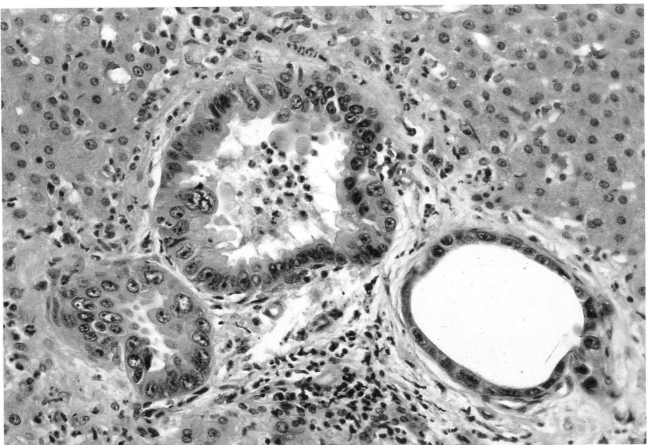

FIGURE 6–80 Colangiocarcinoma in-situ. Cell block prepara-tion showing portal tract adjacent to tumor with colangiocar-cinoma in-situ, a finding diagnostic of bile duct origin. (Hematoxylin & eosin, ×64.)

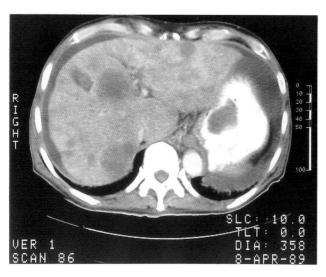

FIGURE 6–81 Angiosarcoma. Computed tomography of the abdomen demonstrating multiple lesions mimicking metastatic disease.

ANGIOSARCOMA

Angiosarcoma (AS) is an extremely rare primary malignancy of the liver that, similar to HCC and CC, occurs principally in older men.[35] Predisposing risk factors include exposure to chemical toxins such as thorotrast,[34] vinyl chloride,[36] and arsenic.[37] Cirrhosis may be present in up to 30 percent of cases.[38] Most patients present with hepatomegaly and multiple lesions mimicking metastatic disease (Figure 6–81).[38]

Grossly, tumor nodules are soft and hemorrhagic, with ill-defined borders (Figure 6–82). Histologically, there are two basic growth patterns:

1. Interdigitating or cystic, composed of sinusoids, often cystically dilated, lined by plump, pleomorphic, hyperchromatic endothelial cells interdigitating between benign hepatic parenchyma (Figure 6–83).
2. Solid, composed of sheets of pleomorphic, hyperchromatic, spindled endothelial cells forming ill-defined vascular spaces (Figure 6–84).

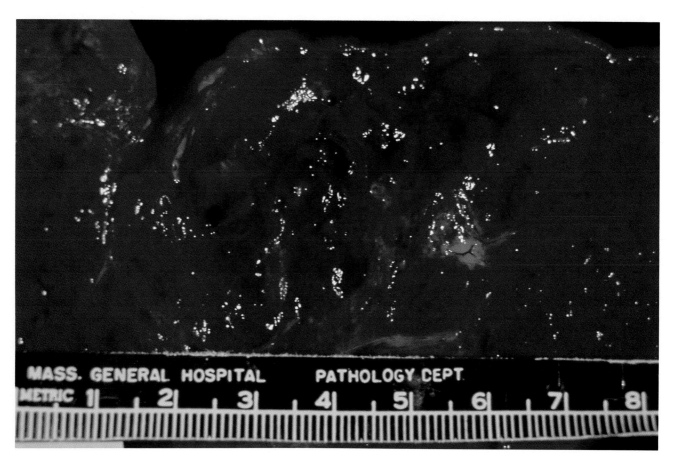

FIGURE 6–82 Angiosarcoma. Tumor nodules are soft and hemorrhagic with ill-defined borders.

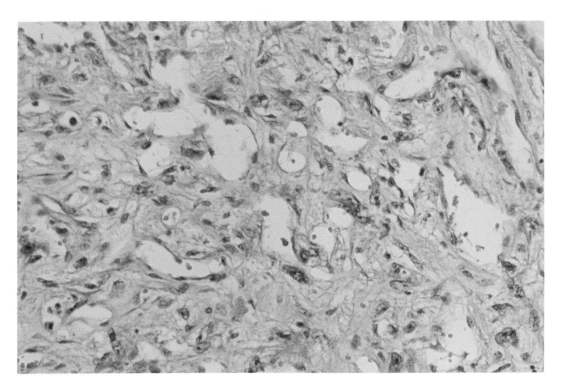

FIGURE 6–83 Angiosarcoma. Interdigitating or cystic growth pattern composed of sinusoids lined by plump, pleomorphic, hyperchromatic endothelial cells interdigitating between benign hepatic parenchyma. (Hematoxylin & eosin, ×64.) (Courtesy of Dr. Robert Young, Massachusetts General Hospital, Boston.)

FIGURE 6–84 Angiosarcoma. Solid growth pattern composed of pleomorphic, hyperchromatic, spindled endothelial cells forming ill-defined vascular spaces. (Hematoxylin & eosin, ×64.)

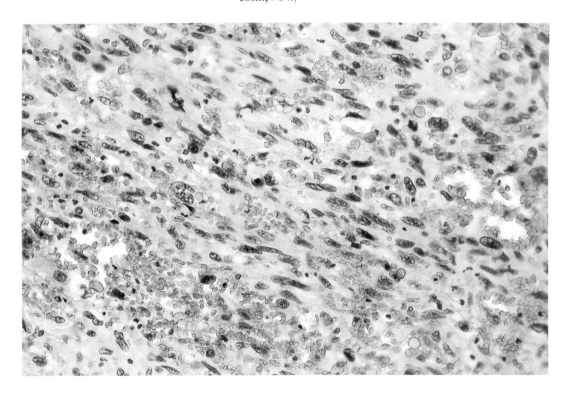

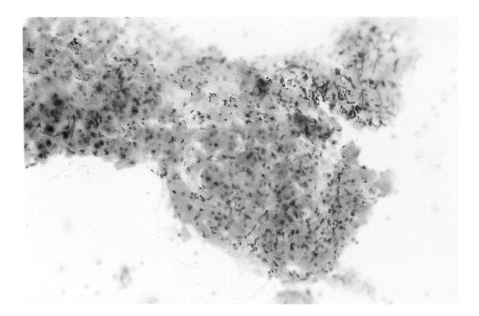

FIGURE 6–85 Angiosarcoma. Fragment of benign hepatocytes with marked bile stasis adjacent to hypercellular fragments of spindle cells. (Hematoxylin & eosin, ×64.)

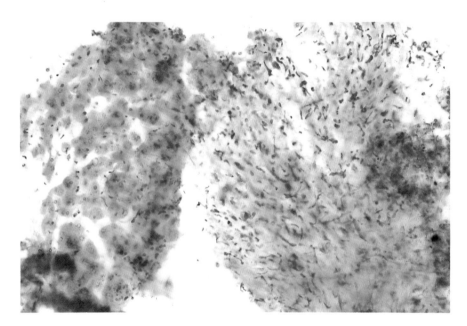

FIGURE 6–86 Angiosarcoma. Large cellular fragment of very hyperchromatic and pleomorphic spindled cells adjacent to benign liver with cholestasis. (Papanicolaou, ×100.)

Aspirate smears of AS with a solid growth pattern produce variably sized cellular fragments of spindle cells that may be adjacent to or associated with benign hepatocytes that may demonstrate cholestasis (Figure 6–85). The cells have obviously malignant characteristics with hyperchromasia and marked pleomorphism of both cell and nuclear size and shape (Figure 6–86). The spindle cell features predominate, but some groups of neoplastic cells may have a more epithelioid appearance.

The differential diagnosis includes other sarcomas such as leiomyosarcoma. Immunocytochemistry for Factor VIII is often necessary for definitive diagnosis. It is important to keep in mind, however, that not all ASs stain positively for Factor VIII, and the staining pattern may be quite focal,[3] so a negative stain does not necessarily rule out the diagnosis of AS.

Aspiration smears of the interdigitating or cystic type of AS show loose groupings of hepatocytic and neoplastic endothelial cells with a more epithelioid rather than spindle cell appearance (Figure 6–87). The nuclei are round to oval with hyperchromasia that may blend into the hepatocytic nuclei, making the cluster of hepatocytes look hypercellular but not necessarily malignant. Less well-differentiated tumors will have smears composed of more anaplastic single cells.[4]

Immunoperoxidase stains showing cells positive for Factor VIII (Figure 6–88) and negative for keratin and CEA support a diagnosis of AS.

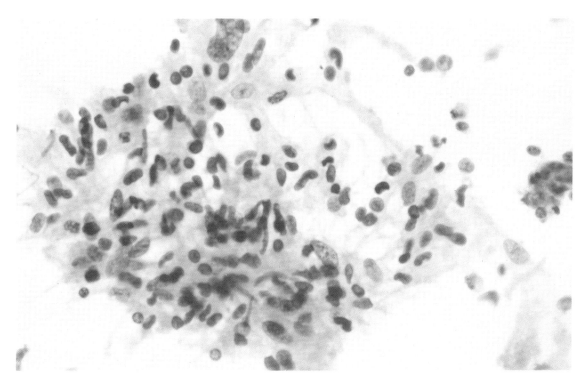

FIGURE 6–87 Angiosarcoma. Aspirate smears of the better differentiated tumors with the cystic or interdigitating growth pattern produce cellular clusters where the malignant endothelial cell nuclei deceivingly blend into those of the hepatocytic nuclei, producing a hypercellular but not necessarily malignant appearance. (Papanicolaou, ×160.)

FIGURE 6–88 Angiosarcoma. Tumor cells are positive for Factor VIII. (Immunoperoxidase, ×160.)

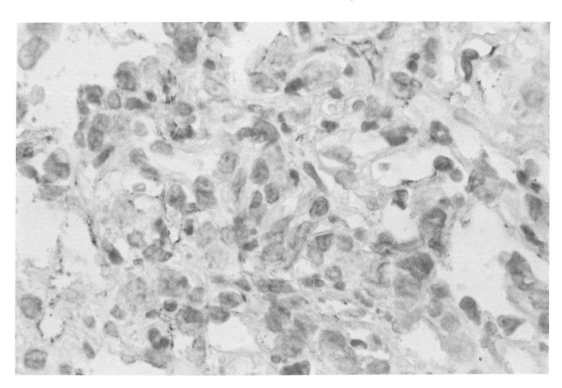

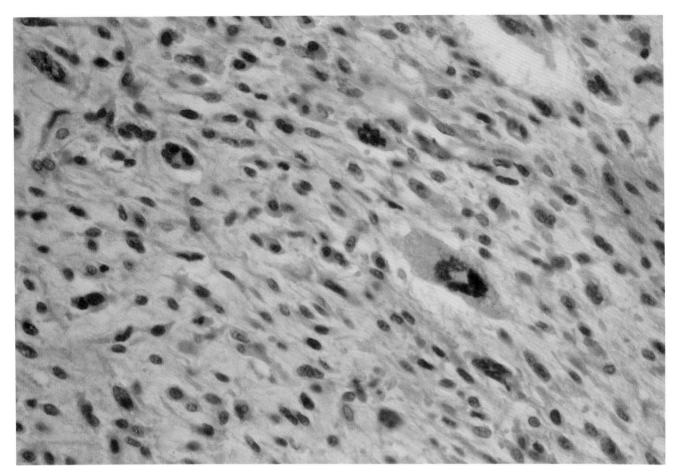

FIGURE 6–89 Embryonal sarcoma. Histologic section demonstrating marked variation in tumor cell size and shape. (Hematoxylin & eosin, ×100.) (Courtesy of Dr. Fiona Graeme-Cook, Massachusetts General Hospital, Boston.)

EMBRYONAL SARCOMA

Embryonal sarcoma (ES), also known as malignant mesenchymona and mesenchymal sarcoma, is an extremely rare neoplasm of children.[39]

Aspiration smears recapitulate the varied histomorphologic patterns within these tumors (Figure 6–89), demonstrating large, markedly anaplastic cells (Figure 6–90), tumor giant cells (Figure 6–91), spindle cells (Figure 6–92), and cells with cytoplasmic globules (Figure 6–93) that stain positively with periodic acid-Schiff after diastase digestion (Figure 6–94).

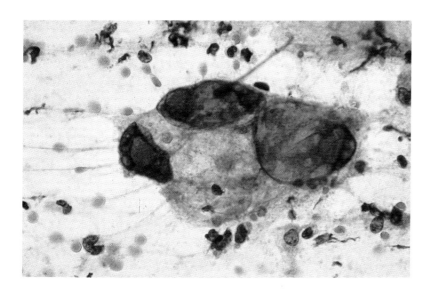

FIGURE 6–90 Embryonal sarcoma. Large anaplastic tumor cells. (Hematoxylin & eosin, ×250.)

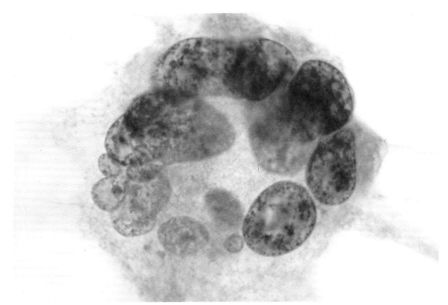

FIGURE 6–91 Embryonal sarcoma. Multinucleated tumor giant cell. (Papanicolaou, ×250.)

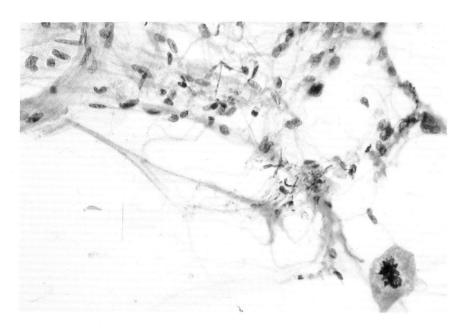

FIGURE 6–92 Embryonal sarcoma. Spindle cell component. (Papanicolaou, ×160.)

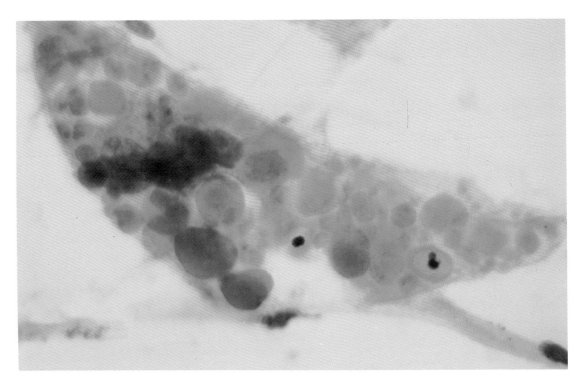

FIGURE 6–93 Embryonal sarcoma. Malignant tumor cells with intracytoplasmic globules. (Papanicolaou, ×250.)

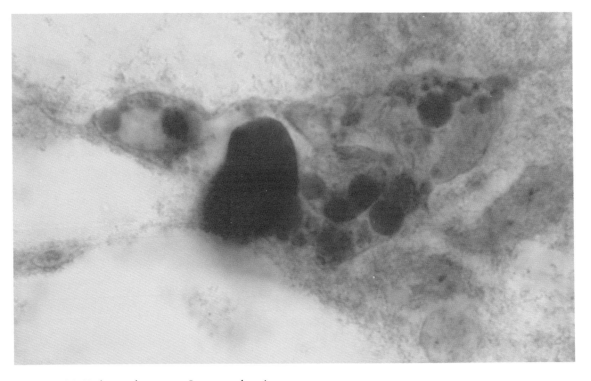

FIGURE 6–94 Embryonal sarcoma. Intracytoplasmic globules stain positively with the periodic acid-Schiff stain and resist diastase digestion. (Periodic acid-Schiff stain with diastase, ×250.)

REFERENCES

1. Munoz N, Bosch X. Epidemiology of hepatocellular carcinoma. In: Okuda K, Ashak KG, eds. Neoplasms of the liver. Tokyo: Springer-Verlag, 1987;3–19.

2. Chen DS. Sung EL. Serum alpha-fetoprotein in hepatocellular carcinoma. Cancer 1977;40:779–783.

3. Kanel CG, Korula J. Atlas of liver pathology. Philadelphia: WB Saunders, 1992;186.

4. Frias-Hidnegi D. Guides to clinical aspiration biopsy: liver and pancreas. New York: Agaku-Shoin, 1988;77.

5. Tao L-C. Transabdominal fine-needle aspiration biopsy. New York: Agaku-Shoin, 1990; 80.

6. Noguchi S, Yamamoto R, Tatsuta M, Kasugai H, Okuda S, Wada A, Tamura H. Cell features and patterns in fine-needle aspiration of hepatocellular carcinoma. Cancer 1986;58:321–328.

7. Pitman MB, Szyfelbein WM. The significance of endothelium in the FNA diagnosis of hepatocellular carcinoma. Diagn Cytopathol (in press).

8. Pedio G, Landolt V, Zobeli L, Gut D. Fine needle aspiration of the liver: Significance of hepatocytic naked nuclei in the diagnosis of hepatocellular carcinoma. Acta Cytol 1988;32:437–442.

9. Johnson DE, Powers CN, Rupp G, Frable WJ. Immunocytochemical staining of fine-needle aspiration biopsies of the liver as a diagnostic tool for hepatocellular carcinoma. Mod Pathol 1992;5:117–123.

10. Roncalli M, Borzio M, De Biagi G, Sevida E, Cantaboni A, Sironi M, Taccagni GL. Liver cell dysplasia and hepatocellular carcinoma: a histological and immunohistochemical study. Histopathol 1985;9:209–221.

11. Buchanan TF, Huvous AG. Clear-cell carcinoma of the liver. A clinicopathologic study of 13 patients. AM J Clin Pathol 1974;61:529–539.

12. Donat EE, Anderson V, Tao L-C. Cytodiagnosis of clear cell hepatocellular carcinoma. A case report. Acta Cytol 1991;35:671–675.

13. Craig JR, Peters RL, Edmondson HA, Masao O. Fibrolamellar carcinoma of the liver. A tumor of adolescents and young adults with distinctive clinocopathologic features. Cancer 1980;46:372–379.

14. Farhi DC, Shikes RH, Murari PJ, Silverberg SG. Hepatocellular carcinoma in young people. Cancer 1983;52:1516–1525.

15. Lack EE, Neane C, Vawter GF. Hepatocellular carcinoma. Review of 32 cases in childhood and adolescence. Cancer 1983;52:1510–1515.

16. Berman MA, Burnham JA, Sheahan DG. Fibrolamellar carcinoma of the liver: An immunohistochemical study of nineteen cases and a review of the literature. Hum Pathol 1988;19:784–794.

17. Paradinas FJ, Melia WM, Wilkinson ML, et al. High serum vitamin B$_{12}$ binding capacity as a marker of the fibrolamellar variant of hepatocellular carcinoma. BMJ 1982;285:840.

18. Greenberg M, Filler RM. Hepatic tumors. In: Pizzo PA, Poplack DG, eds. Principals and practice of pediatric oncology. Philadelphia: JB Lippincott 1989; 569.

19. Asak KG, Glunz PR. Hepatoblastoma and hepatocellular carcinoma in infancy and childhood: report of 45 cases. Cancer 1967;20:396–422.

20. Haas JE, Muczynski KA, Krailo M, Ablin A, Land V, Vietti TJ, Hammond GD. Histopathology and prognosis in childhood hepatoblastoma and hepatocarcinoma. Cancer 1990;64:1082.

21. Gonzalez-Crussi F, Upton MP, Maurer HS. Hepatoblastoma: Attempt at characterization of histologic subtypes. Am J Surg Pathol 1982;6:599–612.

22. Watanabe I. Histopathologic features of liver cell carcinoma in infancy and childhood and their relations to surgical prognosis. Jpn J Cancer Clin 1977;23:691–702.

23. Gonzalez-Crussi F. Undifferentiated small cell ("anaplastic") hepatoblastoma. Pediatr Pathol 1991;11: 155–162.

24. Lack EE, Neane C, Vawter GF. Hepatoblastoma: A clinical and pathologic study of 54 cases. Am J Surg Pathol 1982;6:693–705.

25. Bhatia A, Mehrootra P. Fine needle aspiration cytology in a case of hepatoblastoma. Acta Cytol 1986;30 439–441.

26. Dekmezian R, Sneigi N, Papok S, Ordonez NG. Fine needle aspiration cytology of pediatric patients with primary hepatic tumors. Diagn Cytopathol 1988;4: 162–168.

27. Suen KC. Diagnosis of primary hepatic neoplasm by fine needle aspiration biopsy cytology. Diagn Cytopathol 1986;2:99–109.

28. Wahely PE Jr, Silverman JF, Geisinger KR, Frable WJ. Fine needle aspiration cytology of hepatoblastoma. Mod Pathol 1990;3:688–693.

29. Kaw YT, Hansen K. Fine needle aspiration cytology of undifferentiated small cell ("anaplastic") hepatoblastoma. A case report. Acta Cytol 1993;37: 216–220.

30. Mori W, Nagasako K. Cholangiocarcinoma and related lesion. In: Okuda K, Peters RL, eds. Hepatocellular carcinoma. New York: Wiley, 1976; 227–246.

31. Akwari OE, Van Heerden JA, Foulk WT, et al. Cancer of the bile ducts associated with ulcerative colitis. Ann Surg 1975;181:303–309.

32. Hane PC. The relationship between primary carcinoma of the liver and infestation with *Clonorchis sinensis*. J Pathol Bacteriol 1956;72:239–246.

33. Witlatch S, Nunez C, Pitlik DA. Fine needle aspiration biopsy of the liver. A study of 102 consecutive cases. Acta Cytol 1984;28:719–725.

34. Weinberg CD, Ranchod M. Thorotrast-induced hepatic cholangiocarcinoma and angiosarcoma. Hum Pathol 1979;10:108–112.

35. Locker GY, Doroshow JH, Zwelling LA, et al. The clinical features of hepatic angiosarcoma: a report of four cases and a review of the English literature. Medicine 1979;58:48–64.

36. Thomas LB, Popper H, Berk PD, et al. Vinyl-chloride-induced liver disease. From ideopathic portal hypertension (Banti's syndrome) to angiosarcoma. N Engl J Med 1975;292:17–22.

37. Lander JJ, Stanley RJ, Sumner HW, et al. Angiosarcoma of the liver associated with Fowler's solution (potassium arsenite). Gastroenterology 1975;68:1582–1586.

38. Ludwing J, Hoffman HN II. Hemangiosarcoma of the liver: Spectrum of morphologic changes and clinical findings. Mayo Clinic Proc 1975;50:255–263.

39. Aoyana C, Hachitanda Y, Sato JK, Said JW, Shimada H. Undifferentiated (embryonal) sarcoma of the liver. A tumor of uncertain histogenesis showing divergent differentiation. Am J Surg Pathol 1991;15:615–615.

CHAPTER 7

Metastatic Tumors of the Liver

Martha Bishop Pitman and
Wanda Maria Szyfelbein

The vast majority of malignant tumors in the liver are metastatic, most commonly from the colon, pancreas, breast, and lung in the adult.[1] Likewise, the most common reason for fine needle aspiration biopsy (FNAB) is for the diagnosis of metastatic disease. In most cases the primary tumor is known, making interpretation of the aspirate less difficult. In some cases, however, there is no known primary tumor, and the patient's physician often must rely on the cytopathologist to suggest possible primary sites. Although metastatic tumors tend to have a cytomorphologic appearance in the liver similar to the appearance in the organ of origin, general classifications of tumors, such as adenocarcinomas, look identical in many cases no matter what their primary location. There are certain features of some tumors, however, that are characteristic for their site of origin and, when present, are extremely helpful in suggesting a primary site.

The gross and radiographic presentations of metastatic tumors are generally characterized by multiple rounded nodules with smooth discrete edges (Figure 7–1). It is the radiographic picture at the time of FNAB that often initially suggests a metastasis in cases of unknown primary tumors.

We present a wide array of metastatic tumors, concentrating on the most common followed by less common but not rare tumors and then a couple of rare and unusual tumors that we have encountered.

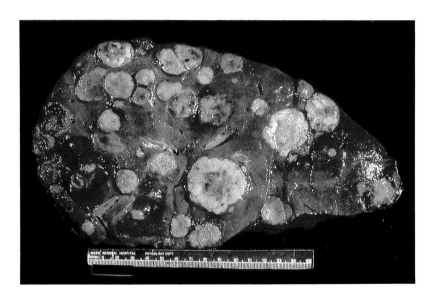

FIGURE 7–1 Multiple rounded nodules characteristic of metastatic tumor. (Courtesy of Dr. Fiona Graeme-Cook, Massachusetts General Hospital, Boston.)

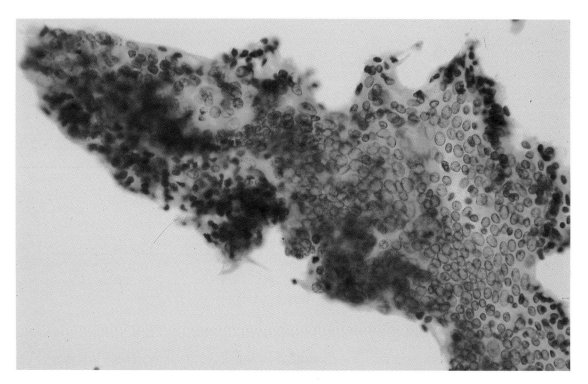

FIGURE 7–2 Metastatic colonic adenocarcinoma. Flat folded sheet with typical glandular honeycombing. (Papanicolaou, ×100.)

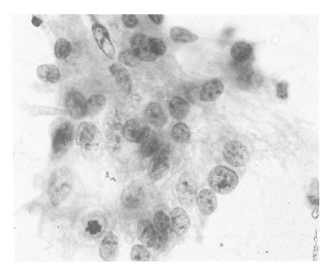

FIGURE 7–3 Metastatic colonic adenocarcinoma. Glandular cells with round to oval nuclei, vesicular chromatin, prominent nuclei, and vacuolated, delicate, lacey cytoplasm. (Papanicolaou, ×250.)

MOST COMMON

Adenocarcinoma

Colon

Colonic adenocarcinoma in the well to moderately differentiated form is composed of columnar cells with oval nuclei with varying degrees of pleomorphism, hyperchromasia, and nucleolar prominence present in flat sheets with typical glandular honeycombing (Figure 7–2) and three-dimensional groups with lacey to vacuolated cytoplasm (Figure 7–3). Characteristic of a colonic origin is the presence of prominent apical cytoplasm illustrating the columnar nature of the cells (Figures 7–4 and 7–5) and, most importantly, the presence of a "dirty," necrotic background (Figure 7–6). Staining artifact can sometimes make the necrotic background appear orangeophilic (Figure 7–7); this should not be mistaken for keratin debris of a squamous cell carcinoma. Cell block preparations may demonstrate the presence of goblet cells (Figure 7–8).

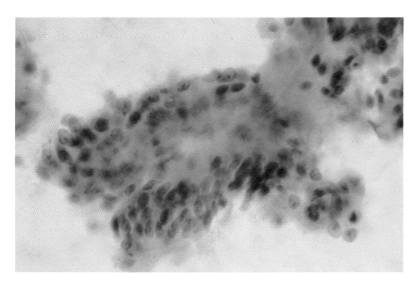

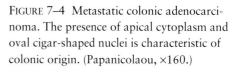

FIGURE 7–4 Metastatic colonic adenocarcinoma. The presence of apical cytoplasm and oval cigar-shaped nuclei is characteristic of colonic origin. (Papanicolaou, ×160.)

FIGURE 7–5 Metastatic colonic adenocarcinoma. Apical cytoplasm characteristic of columnar cells may be present only focally. (Papanicolaou, ×160.)

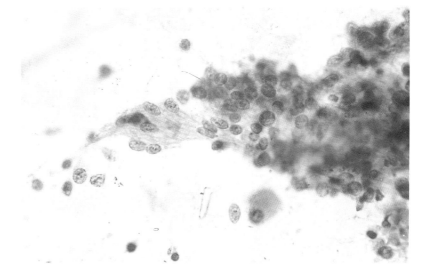

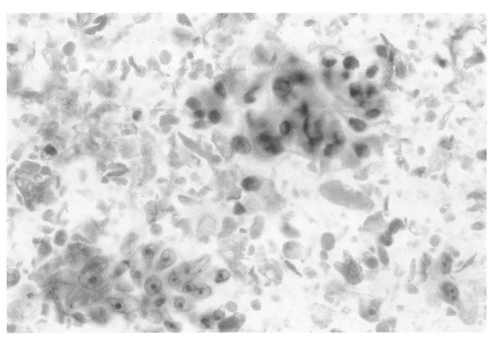

FIGURE 7–6 Metastatic colonic adenocarcinoma. A "dirty" necrotic background is characteristic of colonic origin. (Papanicolaou, ×160.)

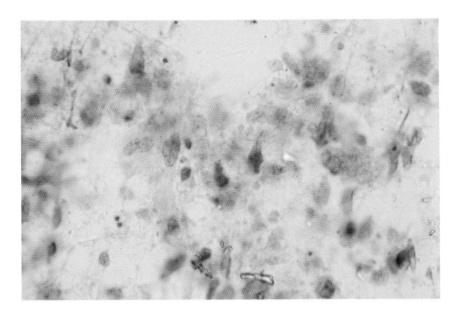

FIGURE 7–7 Metastatic colonic adenocarcinoma. Staining artifact may cause artifactual orangeophilia of necrotic debris, imitating keratin debris in squamous cell carcinoma. (Papanicolaou, ×160.)

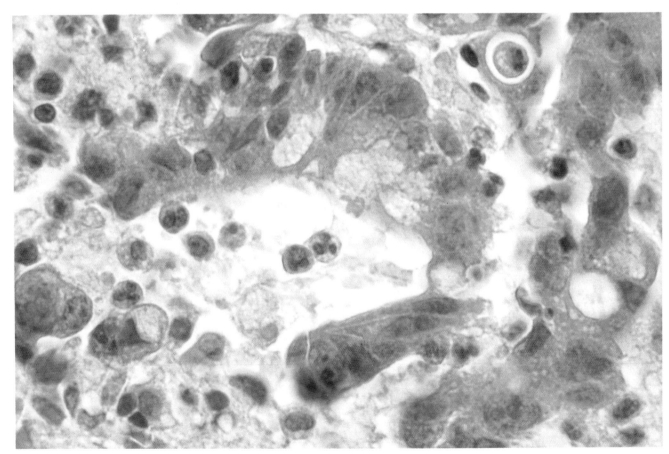

FIGURE 7–8 Metastatic colonic adenocarcinoma. A cell block preparation may demonstrate goblet cells. (Hematoxylin & eosin, ×160.)

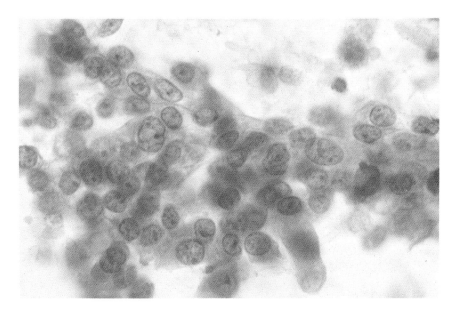

FIGURE 7–9 Metastatic pancreatic adeno-carcinoma. The diagnosis of adenocarci-noma is made by the presence of round to oval vesicular nuclei with nucleoli and delicate cytoplasm. (Hematoxylin & eosin, ×250.)

Pancreas

Pancreatic adenocarcinoma may appear morpho-logically identical to cholangiocarcinoma with groups of cuboidal to columnar cells occurring in nondescript clus-ters easily identified as adenocarcinoma by the presence of delicate cytoplasm and round to oval vesicular nuclei with nucleoli (Figure 7–9). Often seen in tumors of pancre-atic origin is the presence of prominent papillarity (Fig-ures 7–10 and 7–11). Mucin may also be present.

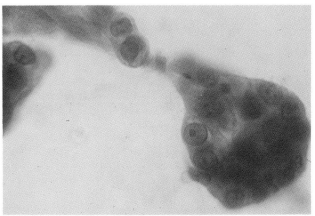

FIGURE 7–10 Metastatic pancreatic adenocarcinoma. Prominent papillarity is often seen in tumors of pancreatic origin. (Hematoxylin & eosin, ×250.)

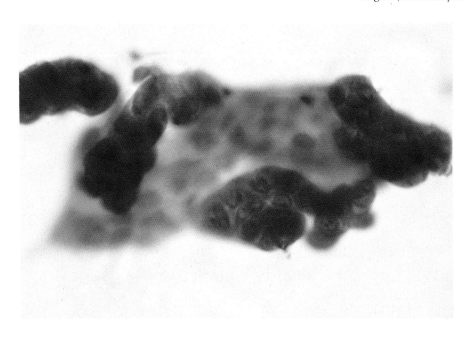

FIGURE 7–11 Metastatic pancreatic adenocarcinoma. The presence of prominent papillarity is not uncommon in tumors of pancreatic origin. (Hematoxylin & eosin, ×160.)

Breast

Adenocarcinoma from the breast, of the typical infiltrating ductal type, has a bland, monomorphous, often low-grade appearance (Figure 7–12). Cells are relatively uniform in size and shape, do not demonstrate marked nuclear atypicality, and may be confused with slightly atypical bile duct epithelium (Figure 7–13). The key to their origin rests in the characteristic smear pattern that aids in the diagnosis of malignancy on breast aspirates—that is, the presence of dishesive groups and single intact cells with eccentrically placed, often cone-shaped, dense cytoplasm and slightly pleomorphic and hyperchromatic nuclei, usually with small but prominent nucleoli (Figure 7–14). These same single intact cells can be seen around the more cohesive clusters of similar cells in the previous two figures. Air-dried May-Grünwald-Giemsa(MGG)–stained slides beautifully demonstrate these cytoplasmic features (Figure 7–15). Small cells lined up in a row with nuclear molding also suggests breast carcinoma and is commonly seen in, but not specific to, carcinomas of lobular origin (Figure 7–16).

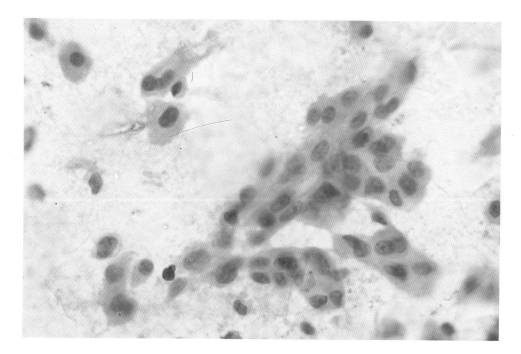

FIGURE 7–12 Metastatic breast carcinoma, infiltrating ductal type. Aspirate smears contain flat, irregular groups with a characteristic low-grade monomorphic glandular appearance. (Papanicolaou, ×100.)

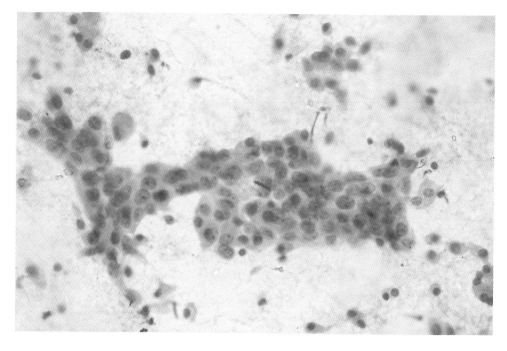

FIGURE 7–13 Metastatic breast carcinoma, infiltrating ductal type. Irregular cluster of bland-appearing cells resembling reactive bile duct epithelium. (Papanicolaou, ×100.)

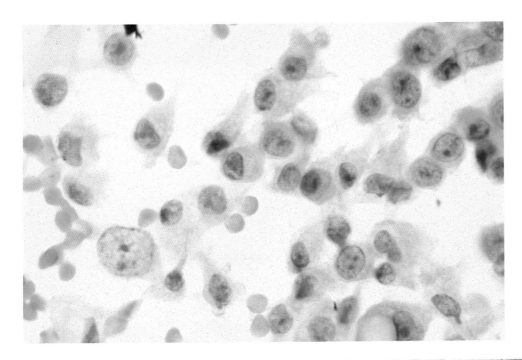

FIGURE 7–14 Metastatic breast carcinoma, infiltrating ductal type. The characteristic smear pattern typical of that in fine needle aspiration biopsy of the breast composed of isolated intact cells with eccentric cone-shaped cytoplasm. (Papanicolaou, ×160.)

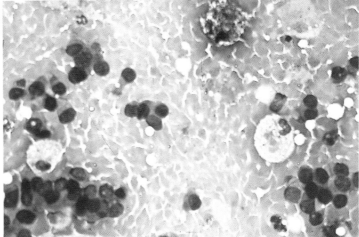

FIGURE 7–15 Metastatic breast carcinoma, infiltrating ductal type. Air-dried smears also demonstrate typical cytoplasmic features with dense cone-shaped appearance. (May-Grünwald-Giemsa, ×100.)

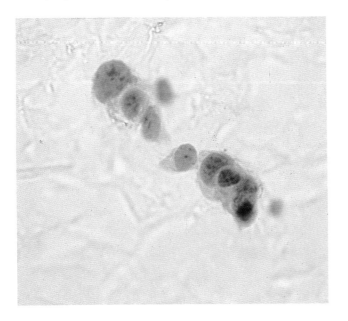

FIGURE 7–16 Metastatic breast carcinoma, lobular type. Malignant cells in single file arrangement with nuclear molding. (Papanicolaou, ×250.)

Lung

Lung adenocarcinomas are diverse in their morphology, ranging from tubular-glandular adenocarcinomas similar to those from the colon, to low-grade tumors (usually of bronchoalveolar type) resembling breast carcinomas, to papillary adenocarcinomas morphologically identical to those from the pancreas. With the routine use of chest x-rays, however, it is rare that primary lung tumors are unknown. The presence of adenosquamous differentiation is not uncommon in the lung, and although not specific to lung origin, the presence of a tumor composed of an adenocarcinoma and malignant keratinized squamous cells indicates that a primary lung tumor should be high in the differential diagnosis (Figures 7–17 and 7–18).

LESS COMMON

Neuroendocrine Tumors

Neuroendocrine tumors of the carcinoid and islet cell type generally are composed of small cells that range from bland, uniform cells to slightly pleomorphic, hyperchromatic cells. They can arise from the lungs, gastrointestinal tract, and pancreaticobiliary system and are often so small that liver metastases are frequently the initial—and sometimes the only—evidence of disease. The production of active substances such as insulin, somatostatin, gastrin, or catecholamines, to name but a few, and demonstration of them either by serologic or immunocytochemical methods support the diagnosis of such a tumor. Without a known primary tumor or demonstra-

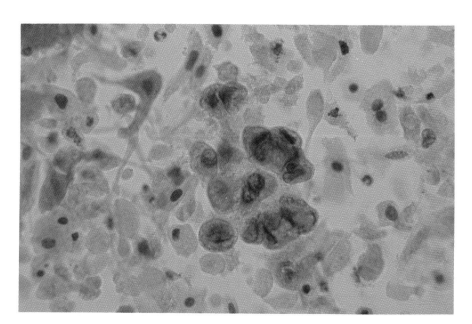

FIGURE 7–17 Metastatic adenosquamous carcinoma of the lung. The tumor is composed of malignant glandular and kerantinized squamous cells. (Papanicolaou, ×160.)

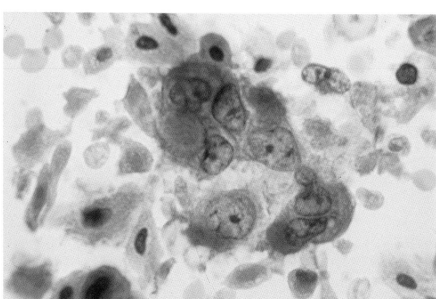

FIGURE 7–18 Metastatic adenosquamous carcinoma of the lung. A special stain for mucin is positive. (Mucicarmine, ×250.)

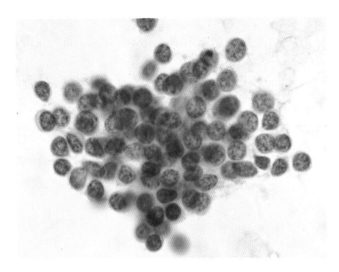

FIGURE 7–19 Metastatic carcinoid tumor. Tumor has an organoid, small nesting smear pattern with a strikingly uniform and monotonous appearance. (Hematoxylin & eosin, ×100.)

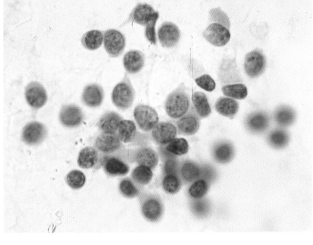

FIGURE 7–20 Metastatic carcinoid tumor. Small, loosely cohesive nest of monotonous uniform cells with delicate, granular cytoplasm. (Papanicolaou, ×250.)

tion of a specific active substance, however, it may be impossible to distinguish between carcinoid and islet cell tumors on cytology alone.

Carcinoid

Carcinoid tumors have an organoid and small nesting smear pattern with a strikingly uniform and monotonous appearance (Figures 7–19 and 7–20). Dishesive groups and single cells are not uncommon (Figure 7–21). The cells have round to oval nuclei, scant delicate and often granular cytoplasm, and a distinctly coarse "salt and pepper" chromatin pattern (Figure 7–22). The smearing of the tumor often destroys this delicate cytoplasm, creating a granular background. Mitotic figures are rare.

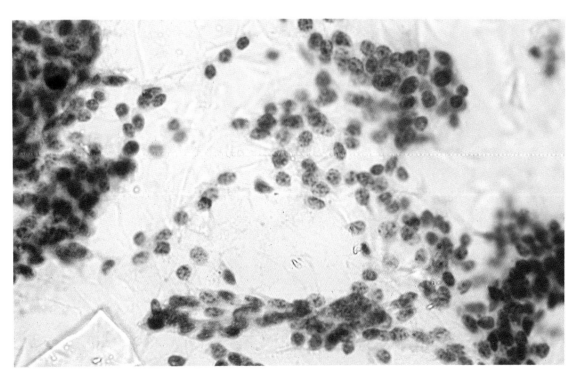

FIGURE 7–21 Metastatic carcinoid tumor. Dishesive groups and single cells are not uncommon. (Papanicolaou, ×250.)

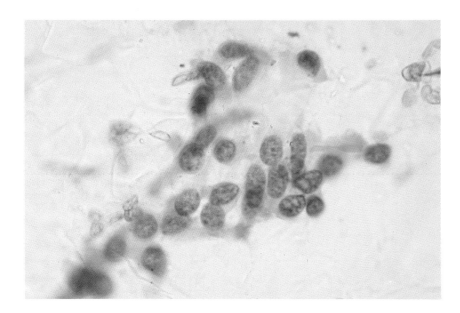

FIGURE 7–22 Metastatic carcinoid tumor. The cells have round to oval nuclei, scant, delicate cytoplasm, and a distinctly coarse "salt and pepper" chromatin pattern. (Papanicolaou, ×250.)

Islet Cell

Islet cell tumors (ICTs) tend to produce a less packeted and organoid smear pattern than carcinoid tumors, occurring more in loose groups (Figure 7–23) and angulated flat sheets (Figure 7–24) and as single cells (Figure 7–25). The cells more often display greater pleomorphism of both cell and nuclear size and shape and contain more abundant, typically eccentric cytoplasm than carcinoid tumors, resulting in a "plasmacytoid" appearance (Figure 7–26). Often ICTs have a less pronounced "salt and pepper" chromatin pattern and may contain prominent nucleoli (Figure 7–27).

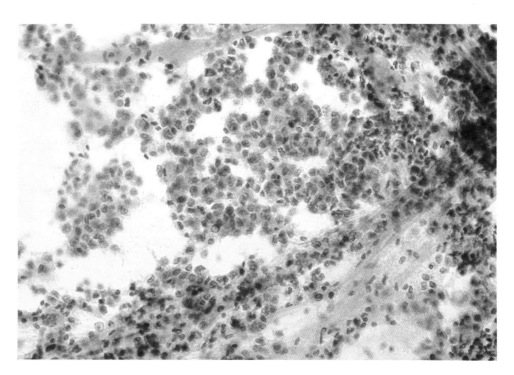

FIGURE 7–23 Metastatic islet cell tumor. Loose clusters and nests of tumor cells. (Papanicolaou, ×100.)

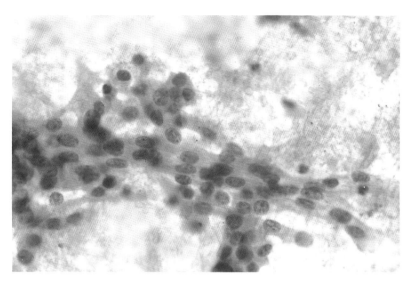

FIGURE 7–24 Metastatic islet cell tumor. Flat, angulated sheet of uniform tumor cells with visible cytoplasm. (Papanicolaou, ×250.)

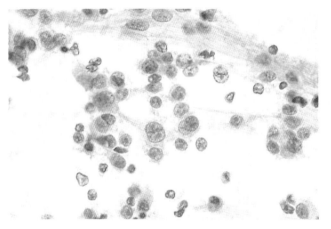

FIGURE 7–25 Metastatic islet cell tumor. Single cells with pleomorphic nuclei, nucleoli, and visible cytoplasm. (Papanicolaou, ×250.)

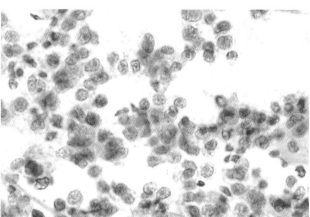

FIGURE 7–26 Metastatic islet cell tumor. Dishesive sheets and single cells with eccentric nuclei, visible cytoplasm, and plasmacytoid appearance. (Papanicolaou, ×250.)

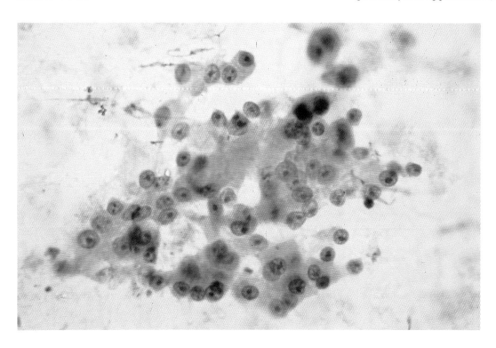

FIGURE 7–27 Metastatic islet cell tumor. The coarse "salt and pepper" neuroendocrine chromatin pattern is less pronounced than in carcinoid tumors, and nucleoli are often prominent. (Papanicolaou, ×250.)

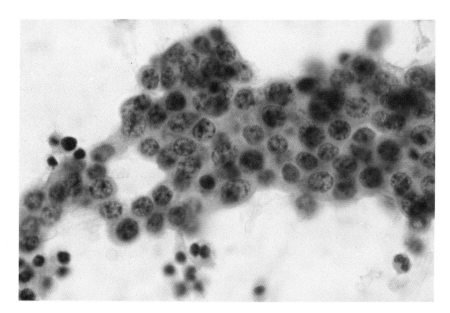

FIGURE 7–28 Neuroendocrine tumor: carcinoid versus islet cell tumor. Uniform organoid arrangement of cells with round nuclei, coarse "salt and pepper" chromatin, and granular cytoplasm. (Papanicolaou, ×250.)

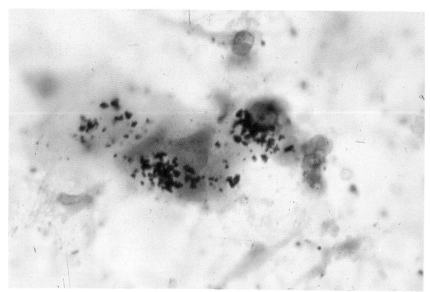

FIGURE 7–29 Neuroendocrine tumor cells demonstrating neurosecretory granules by special stain. (Grimelius, ×250.)

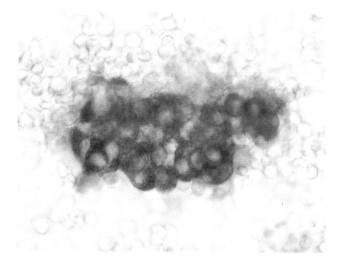

FIGURE 7–30 Neuroendocrine tumor demonstrating chromagranin positivity. (Immunoperoxidase, ×250.)

None of these features, however, are specific. It is virtually impossible to definitively diagnose either of these entities with exclusion of the other with any certainty on cytology alone. Often these features merge, yielding small, uniform cells in organoid packets, flat sheets, and singly with visible cytoplasm, granular "salt and pepper" chromatin, and scattered nucleoli (Figure 7–28). Both carcinoid tumors and ICTs stain positively with a Grimelius stain (Figure 7–29) and demonstrate chromagranin positivity with immunoperoxidase stain (Figure 7–30). Immunocytochemistry performed to identify active substances is often cumbersome and difficult unless a cell block is available with sufficient material to use for the numerous stains. In these cases, we often make a diagnosis of neuroendocrine tumor with both carcinoid and ICT in the differential diagnosis.

Lymphoma

Involvement of the liver by non-Hodgkin's lymphoma rarely may be primary,[2] but in the vast majority of cases the liver is secondarily involved with spleen and/or abdominal lymph nodes almost always affected.[1] Diffuse involvement is more common, but approximately 25 percent of patients will present with irregular multiple or solitary nodules.[3]

Most lymphomas involving the liver are large-cell type[3] and produce a characteristic smear pattern of a diffuse, monomorphous, single-cell population of atypical lymphoid cells (Figure 7–31). Their lymphoid origin is indicated by (1) their dishesive, single nature; (2) their scant cytoplasm; (3) their open nuclei with peripheral clumped chromatin and prominent nucleoli; and (4) the presence of lymphoglandular bodies in the background (Figure 7–32). Lymphoglandular bodies are globules of stripped cytoplasm forming "blue blobs" in the smear background that are best seen on an air-dried MGG stain but are also identified on Papanicolaou (Pap) stains. This artifact of preparation is present in both neoplastic and non-neoplastic lymphoid smears.[4,5] Occasionally uneven smearing will cause lymphocytes to clump in "pseudo-groups" (Figure 7–33), suggesting an epithelial origin. Close examination, however, will demonstrate that the groups are composed of the same cells that are diffusely and singly scattered in the background. This and other features typical of lymphoma should facilitate the correct diagnosis. Cell block preparations (Figure 7–34) are usually very helpful, particularly with respect to supplying tissue for immunoperoxidase studies if needed.

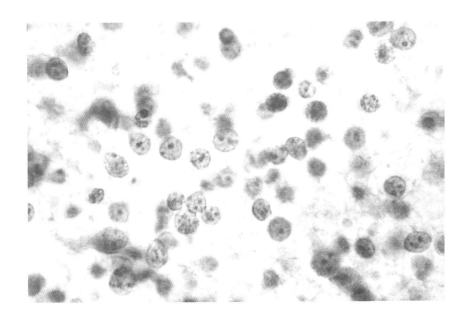

FIGURE 7–31 Metastatic lymphocytic lymphoma, large cell type. Characteristic smear pattern composed of single atypical lymphoid cells with peripherally clumped chromatin, prominent nucleoli, and scant to invisible cytoplasm. (Papanicolaou, ×250.)

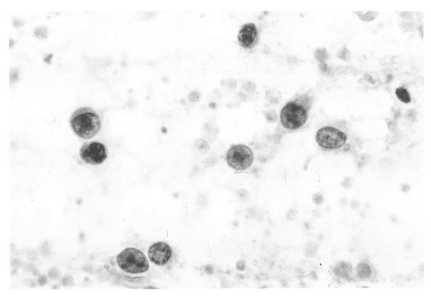

FIGURE 7–32 Metastatic lymphocytic lymphoma, large cell type. Single malignant cells in a background of lymphoglandular bodies, a diagnostic clue that their origin is lymphoid. (Papanicolaou, ×250.)

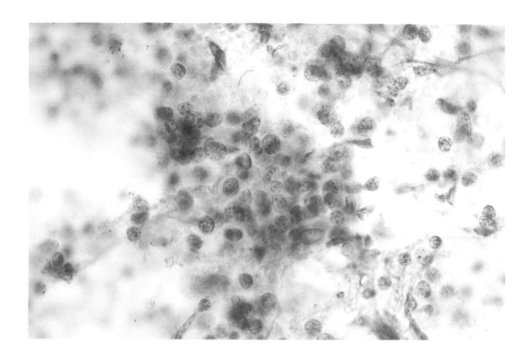

FIGURE 7–33 Metastatic lymphocytic lymphoma, large cell type. Pseudo-group formation may simulate carcinoma. (Papanicolaou, ×160.)

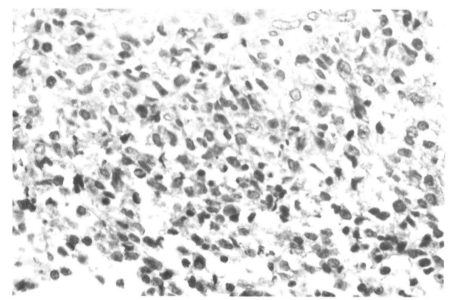

FIGURE 7–34 Metastatic lymphocytic lymphoma, large cell type. Cell block preparation provides easily accessible tissue for special studies.

Small-cell lymphomas prove the most challenging on FNAB. Immunoperoxidase studies are almost always needed. Small, mature lymphocytes with scattered larger atypical lymphoid cells (Figure 7–35) may be seen in a number of reactive processes in the liver. Confirmation of a monoclonal population of lymphocytes (Figures 7–36 through 7–38), however, is diagnostic of malignant lymphoma.

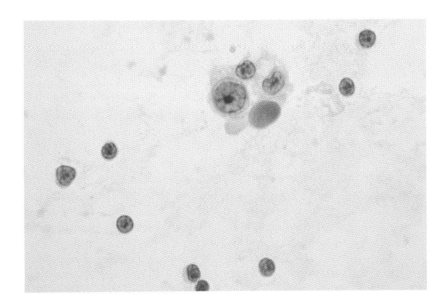

FIGURE 7–35 Metastatic lymphocytic lymphoma, small cell type. Cytospin preparation demonstrating pleomorphic small and larger atypical lymphocytes resembling a reactive process. (Papanicolaou, ×250.)

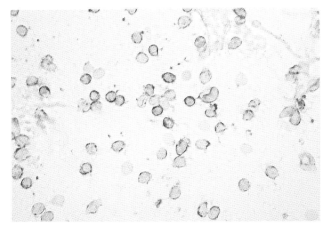

FIGURE 7–36 Metastatic lymphocytic lymphoma, small cell type. Cytospin preparation demonstrating diffuse immunoglobulin M heavy-chain production. (Immunoperoxidase, ×160.)

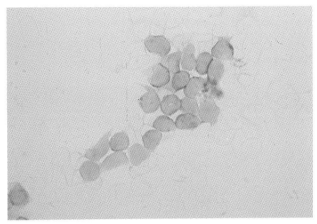

FIGURE 7–37 Metastatic lymphocytic lymphoma, small cell type. Cytospin preparation demonstrating numerous cells positive for kappa-light chain. (Immunoperoxidase, ×250.)

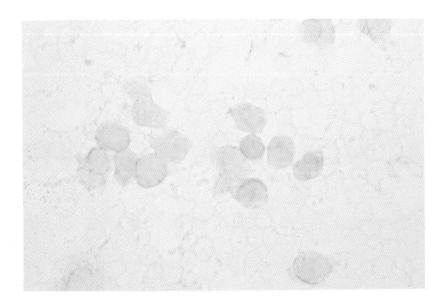

FIGURE 7–38 Metastatic lymphocytic lymphoma, small cell type. Cytospin preparation with no cells positive for lambda-light chain. (Immunoperoxidase, ×250.)

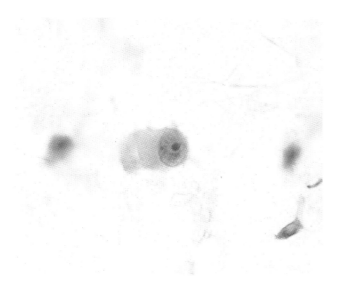

FIGURE 7–39 Metastatic malignant melanoma. Classic melanoma cell with eccentric nucleus and prominent eosinophilic macronucleus. (Papanicolaou, ×250.)

Melanoma

The liver is a frequent site for metastases for melanoma, occurring in approximately 50 percent of patients.[1] Except in cases of classic adenocarcinoma, melanoma should always be considered in the differential diagnosis of solid tumors due to its incredible ability to mimic so may other types of tumors. The classic melanoma cell (Figure 7–39) is a single cell with an eccentric, large, hyperchromatic nucleus containing a prominent, eosinophilic macronucleolus. Intranuclear inclusions (Figure 7–40) are common and pigment may be absent, focal (Figure 7–41), or prominent (Figure 7–42). The presence of melanin pigment is virtually diagnostic, but its nature should be confirmed with a Fontana-Masson stain (Figure 7–43) particularly if scant and there is no history of melanoma, as other epithelial tumors metastatic to the liver may phagocytize a variety of pigments,[2] and bile pigment in atypical, reactive, or neoplastic hepatocytes can mimic melanoma. Cytologists generally recognize four variants of melanoma,[6,7] which may appear as the only cell type or one of a mixture of cell types in a single tumor.[8]

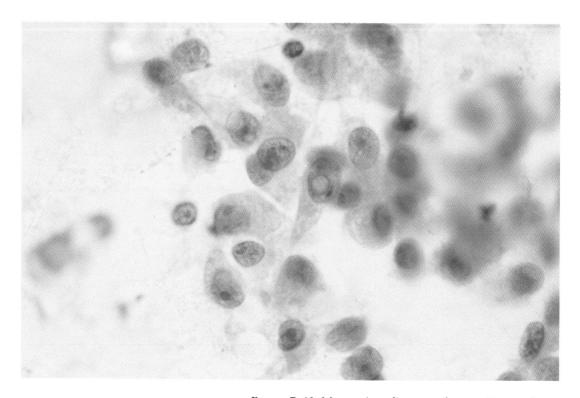

FIGURE 7–40 Metastatic malignant melanoma. Intranuclear inclusions are typical of this tumor type. (Papanicolaou, ×250.)

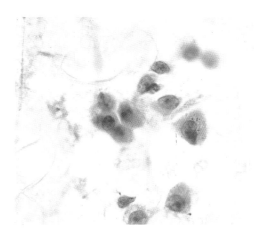

FIGURE 7–41 Metastatic malignant melanoma. Cytoplasmic pigment may be very focal. (Papanicolaou, ×250.)

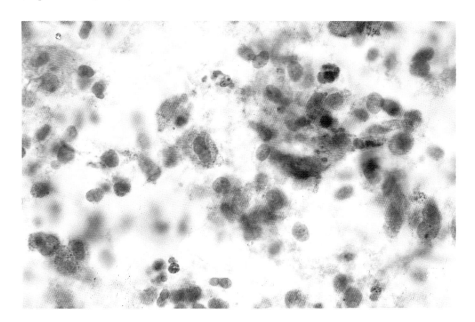

FIGURE 7–42 Metastatic malignant melanoma. Intracytoplasmic pigment may be very prominent. (Papanicolaou, ×250.)

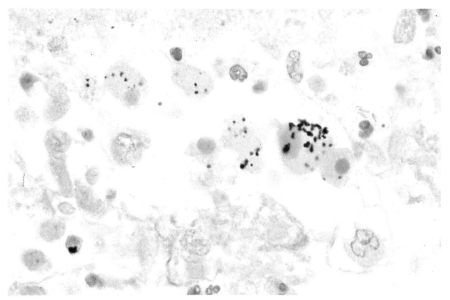

FIGURE 7–43 Metastatic malignant melanoma. A special stain confirms the identity of intracytoplasmic pigment as melanin. (Fontana-Masson, ×250.)

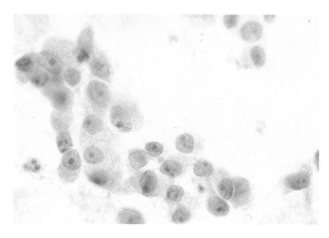

FIGURE 7–44 Metastatic malignant melanoma, epithelial cell type. Clusters of cells with a polygonal shape may resemble carcinoma. This type most closely resembles hepatocellular carcinoma. (Papanicolaou, ×250.)

Epithelial Cell Type

The epithelial cell type (Figure 7–44) consists predominantly of single cells like those described above for the classic melanoma cell, but also contain some cohesive groups resembling a carcinoma. This type is the most easily confused with hepatocellular carcinoma (HCC). Features in common include eosinophilic macronucleoli, intranuclear inclusions, and dense, eosinophilic cytoplasm that may contain pigment. Of course, with HCC the pigment is bile and with melanoma the pigment is melanin. Although these pigments can usually be distinguished on routine stains alone—bile is golden, green, globular, and somewhat refractile (see Chapter 4), and melanin, although variable in size, is usually small and round and typically dark brown to black. When scant, special stains are often necessary to differentiate the two. Cellular dishesiveness and nuclear eccentricity are also

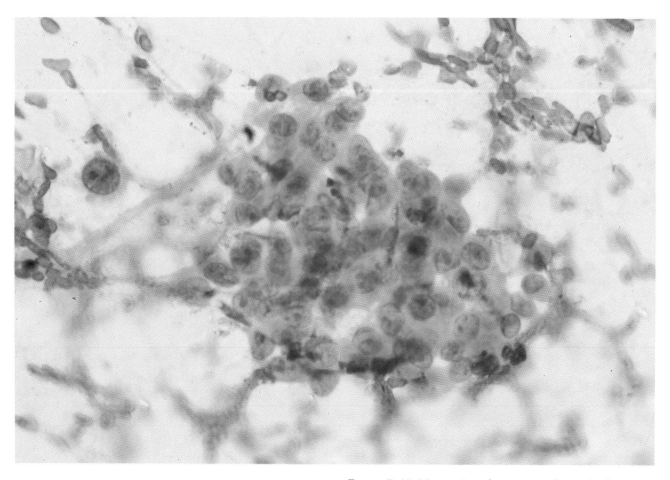

FIGURE 7–45 Metastatic melanoma, small round cell type. Small malignant cells with scant cytoplasm and indistinct nucleoli may mimic other small round cell tumors. (Papanicolaou, ×160.)

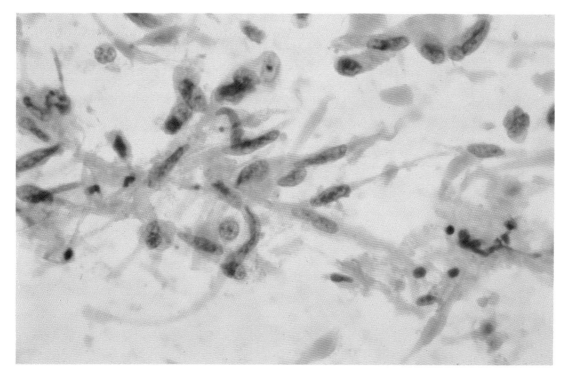

FIGURE 7–46 Malignant melanoma, spindle cell type. This type of melanoma mimics sarcomas and spindle cell neuroendocrine tumors such as carcinoid tumor. (Papanicolaou, ×160.)

much more characteristic of melanoma, and cell clusters are more common, regular, and often associated with either peripheral or transgressing endothelium in HCC (see Chapter 6).

Small Round Cell Type

The small round cell type of melanoma (Figure 7–45) occurs as single cells and groups that can mimic other small round cell tumors, particularly non-Hodgkin's lymphoma and small cell undifferentiated carcinoma. As previously mentioned, smear artifact can cause pseudo-group formation in lymphoma, but this is an infrequent finding in lymphoma, whereas group formation in melanoma is much more common. Also, the presence of eosinophilic macronucleoli, intranuclear inclusions, and distinctly visible, well-defined, albeit often scant, cytoplasm are features supportive of melanoma. These features are more apparent on single cells. Small cell carcinoma should display a coarse "salt and pepper" chromatin pattern and some nuclear molding.

Spindle Cell Type

The spindle cell type of melanoma (Figure 7–46) occurs in tight sheets, loose groups, and single cells that have oval nuclei with rounded ends, frequent nuclear grooves, and bipolar cytoplasm. Nucleoli are typically small and dark and intranuclear inclusions infrequent. The primary tumors in the differential diagnosis are neuroendocrine tumors, particularly carcinoid tumors, and mesenchymal sarcomas.

The chromatin pattern in this type of melanoma, although coarse, does not have a clumpy neuroendocrine, "salt and pepper" appearance. Nucleoli that are typical of ICTs are not a feature of spindle cell melanoma. In addition, the pleomorphism and hyperchromasia of spindle cell melanoma is more than would be expected in most spindle cell carcinoids.

Mesenchymal sarcomas tend to occur more often in tight groups with few single cells as opposed to this variant of melanoma, which frequently occurs as loose groups and single cells. Also, sarcomas are less likely to be occult, and a present or previous clinical history of a sarcoma is often known.

Pleomorphic, Large Cell Type

The pleomorphic, large cell type of melanoma is composed of single giant cells with one or more markedly pleomorphic and hyperchromatic nuclei with very irregular borders (Figure 7–47) and resembles other large cell, anaplastic tumors such as large cell undifferentiated carcinoma of the lung, pleomorphic carcinoma of the pancreas, and high-grade sarcomas. Again, history is very helpful in the differential diagnosis of this type. Eosinophilic macronucleoli, intranuclear inclusions, fre-

quent binucleation, and eccentric cytoplasm are all features supportive of melanoma.

In all types of melanoma, however, and particularly in cases where there is no known primary tumor or where characteristic melanin pigment is not present, the diagnosis may be confirmed with immunoperoxidase studies. Melanomas are classically positive for vimentin, neuron-specific enolase, S-100, and HMB-45 (Figure 7–48) and negative for keratin and epithelial membrane antigen.[9,10]

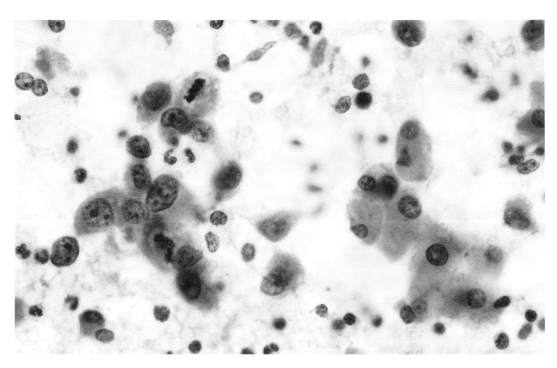

FIGURE 7–47 Metastatic melanoma. Cell block preparation demonstrating positivity for HMB-45. (Immunoperoxidase, ×40.)

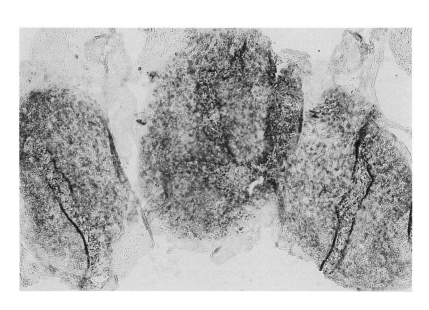

FIGURE 7–48 Metastatic squamous cell carcinoma. The presence of malignant keratinized cells make the diagnosis easy. (Papanicolaou, ×250.)

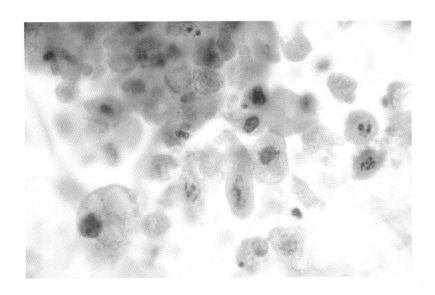

FIGURE 7–49 Metastatic squamous cell carcinoma. The presence of malignant keratinized cells make the diagnosis easy. (Papanicolaou, × 250.)

Squamous Cell Carcinoma

Squamous cell carcinoma (SCC) is relatively easy to diagnose when it is well differentiated enough to produce keratinized cells that stain orangeophilic with Pap stain (Figure 7–49). Less well differentiated tumors in which keratin is not apparent are diagnosed on the basis of their nuclear and cytoplasmic features. The nuclei are generally very pleomorphic and hyperchromatic, with prominent nuclear envelope irregularities and generally no nucleoli; the cytoplasm is dense and abundant (Figure 7–50). Tadpole cells are also characteristic of SCC (Figure 7–51). Poorly differentiated SCC poses the greatest diagnostic difficulty. These tumors can occur in three-dimensional groups (Figure 7–52) and have prominent nucleoli and lacey-appearing cytoplasm due to degeneration (Figure 7–53) mimicking adenocarcinoma. A diagnosis of "poorly differentiated carcinoma, large cell type" is sufficient in this type of case.

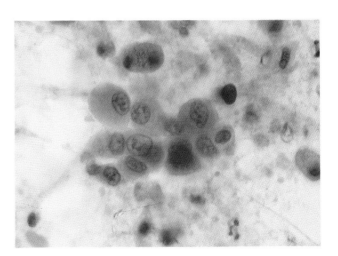

FIGURE 7–50 Metastatic squamous cell carcinoma. These cells have irregular pleomorphic nuclei with nuclear membrane irregularities, no nucleoli, and dense cytoplasm. (Hematoxylin & eosin, ×250.)

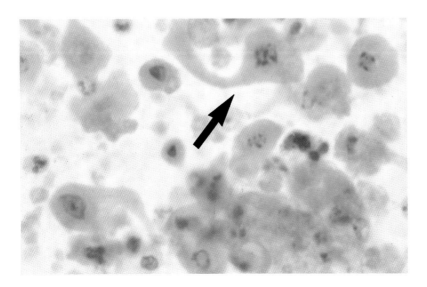

FIGURE 7–51 Metastatic squamous cell carcinoma. Tadpole cells (*arrow*) are characteristic of squamous cell origin. (Papanicolaou, ×250.)

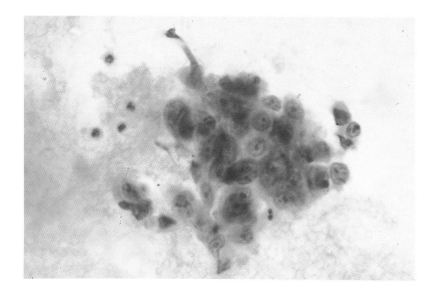

FIGURE 7–52 Metastatic squamous cell carcinoma. Poorly differentiated tumors may occur in clusters resembling adenocarcinoma. (Papanicolaou, ×160.)

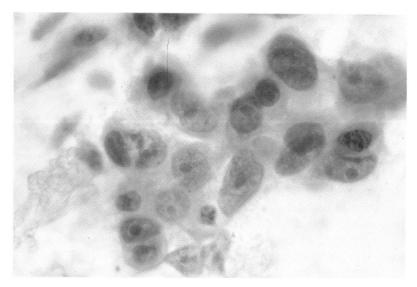

FIGURE 7–53 Metastatic squamous cell carcinoma. Poorly differentiated tumors may also have cells with prominent nucleoli and degenerated lacey-appearing cytoplasm mimicking adenocarcinoma. (Papanicolaou, ×250.)

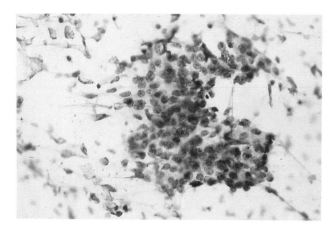

FIGURE 7–54 Metastatic small cell carcinoma. Characteristic clusters of crowded small cells with smear artifact. (Papanicolaou, ×100.)

Small Cell Undifferentiated Carcinoma

Small cell undifferentiated carcinoma occurs predominantly in irregular clusters rather than as single cells and is composed of delicate cells susceptible to smear artifact (Figure 7–54), which is actually a helpful characteristic feature. The nuclei are generally round, with coarsely clumped, "salt and pepper" chromatin and scant cytoplasm (Figure 7–55). Nuclear molding is a prominent feature (Figure 7–56), and abundant necrosis is common. Although nuclear detail is not well demonstrated on an air-dried MGG stain, the small cell size and nuclear molding is easily appreciated (Figure 7–57). These features are characteristic of small cell undifferentiated carcinoma no matter what its origin, and thus are diagnostic of the tumor type but not the tumor origin.

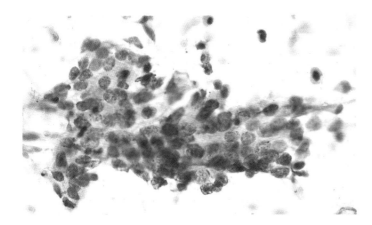

FIGURE 7–55 Metastatic small cell carcinoma. Cells are small with round to oval nuclei, coarse "salt and pepper" chromatin, and scant cytoplasm. (Papanicolaou, ×160.)

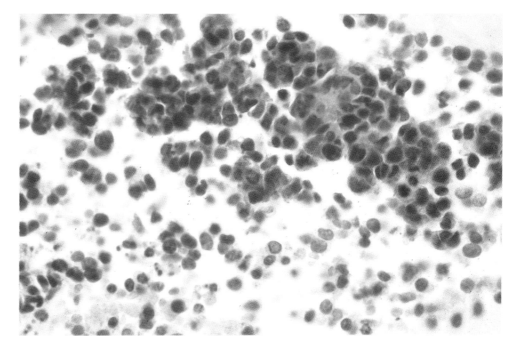

FIGURE 7–56 Metastatic small cell carcinoma. Nuclear molding is characteristic of this tumor type. (Hematoxylin& eosin, ×160.)

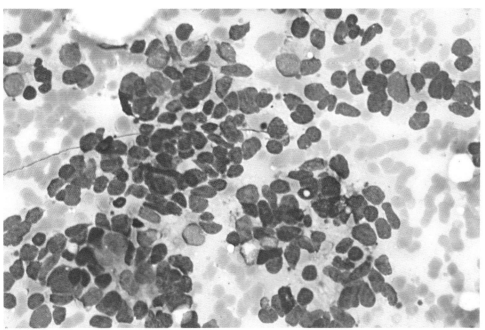

FIGURE 7–57 Metastatic small cell carcinoma. Air-dried smear preparation allows for easy recognition of small cell size and nuclear molding, despite obscuring nuclear chromatin pattern. (May-Grünwald-Giemsa, ×100.)

Renal Cell Carcinoma

Renal cell carcinoma (RCC) is most often of the clear cell type, occasionally the granular cell type, and rarely the spindle cell variant. It is a tumor that very closely resembles HCC (see Chapter 6). Both HCC and granular RCC have round central nuclei, prominent macronucleoli, and granular cytoplasm (Figure 7–58). Renal cell carcinoma, however, more often has a perinucleolar halo—hence the name "owl's eye" nucleus (Figure 7–59). The clear cell variant of HCC and clear cell RCC also have similar nuclear and cytoplasmic features (Figure 7–60). Although RCC a vascular tumor, in our experience, endothelial cells are not present in the distinctive peripheral or transgressing patterns described for HCC.[11] (See Chapter 6.) Morphologic differences are often subtle and sometimes indistinguishable, with clinical evaluation ruling out the presence of an RCC often the only means of distinguishing the two.

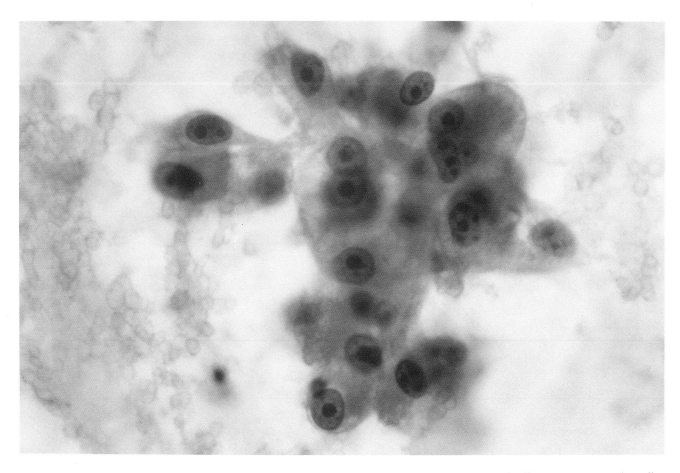

FIGURE 7–58 Metastatic renal cell carcinoma, granular cell type. Cells are polygonal with round central nuclei, prominent nucleoli, and granular cytoplasm mimicking hepatocellular carcinoma. (Hematoxylin & eosin, ×160.)

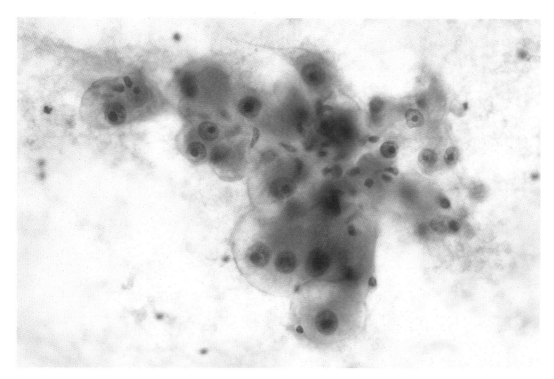

FIGURE 7–59 Metastatic renal cell carcinoma, clear cell type. Cells are polygonal with round central nuclei, prominent nucleoli, and clear vacuolated cytoplasm mimicking hepatocellular carcinoma, clear cell type. (Papanicolaou, ×100.)

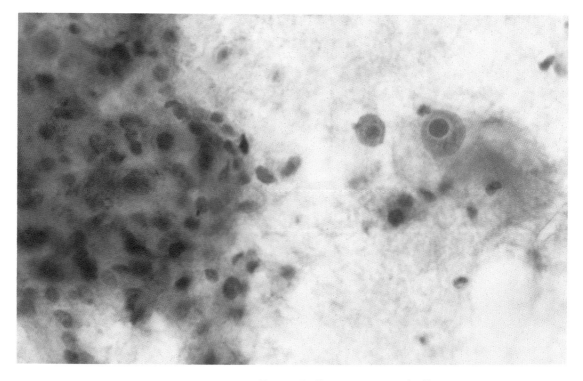

FIGURE 7–60 Metastatic renal cell carcinoma. Characteristic tumor cell with classic "owl's eye" nucleus manifested by prominent eosinophilic macronucleus surrounded by clear halo. (Papanicolaou, ×160.)

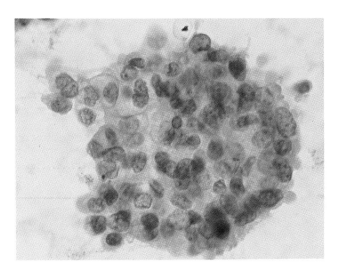

FIGURE 7–61 Metastatic prostate carcinoma. Cells occur in cohesive nests and are composed of somewhat regular round polygonal cells with irregular hyperchromatic overlapping nuclei and clear cytoplasm. (Papanicolaou, ×100.)

Prostatic Carcinoma

Carcinomas of the prostate have a relatively characteristic appearance. Smears are composed of nests (Figure 7–61) and flat sheets (Figure 7–62) of crowded round to polygonal cells with irregular, hyperchromatic, overlapping nuclei, open vesicular chromatin, and small but prominent nucleoli. The cytoplasm is clear with distinct borders (Figure 7–63). Despite the atypicality, the cells have a rather uniform appearance. Other carcinomas with clear cytoplasm are in the differential diagnosis. The high specificity and sensitivity of prostate-specific antigen (Figure 7–64) and prostatic acid phosphatase (Figure 7–65) immunoperoxidase stains are very helpful in making an accurate diagnosis.

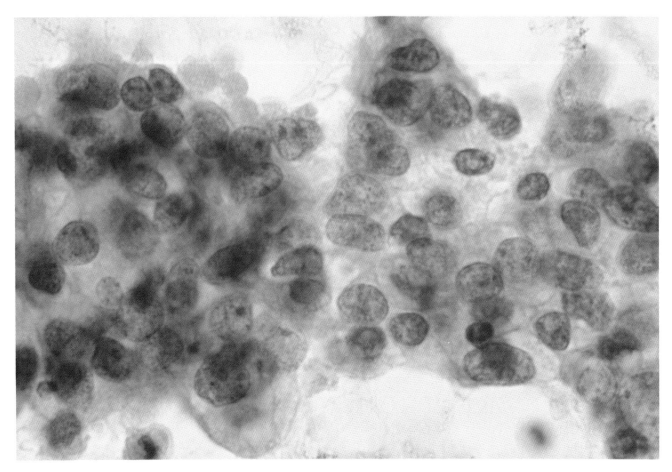

FIGURE 7–62 Metastatic prostate carcinoma. Tumor cells occur in flat sheets and are composed of round polygonal cells with crowded, irregular, overlapping nuclei and clear cytoplasm. (Papanicolaou, ×160.)

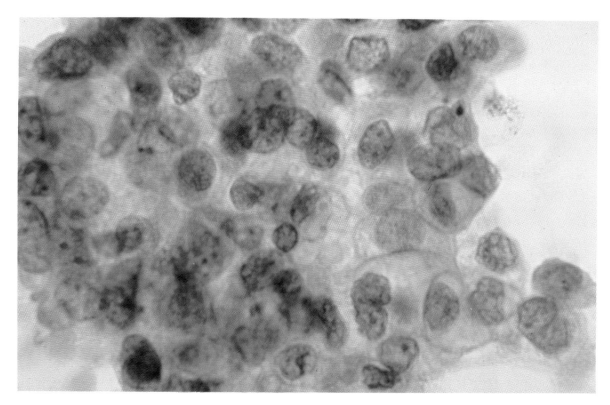

FIGURE 7–63 Metastatic prostate carcinoma. Tumor cells
are relatively uniform with round to oval nuclei, nuclear
membrane irregularities, and clear cytoplasm with focally
distinct borders. Nucleoli may not be conspicuous.
(Papanicolaou, ×250.)

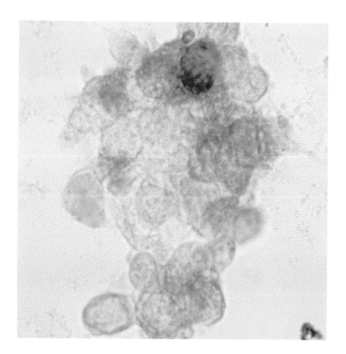

FIGURE 7–64 Metastatic prostate carcinoma. Tumor cells
are positive for prostate-specific antigen. (Immunoperoxidase, ×250.)

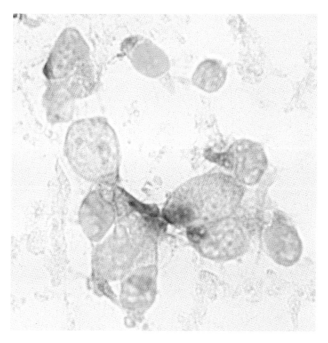

FIGURE 7–65 Metastatic prostate carcinoma. Tumor cells
will be positive for prostatic acid phosphatase. (Immunoperoxidase, ×250.)

Leiomyosarcoma

In our experience, leiomyosarcoma is the most common sarcoma metastatic to the liver. They are very rarely primary neoplasms.[1,12] Grossly, metastatic nodules are typically large and bulky with broad, pushing borders (Figure 7–66). On aspirate smears, cellular clusters of spindle cells (Figure 7–67) predominate, with scattered single cells best illustrating the oval, cigar-shaped nuclei with rounded ends and bipolar cytoplasm (Figure 7–68). Epithelioid features (Figure 7–69) manifested by a polygonal cell shape and round to oval central nuclei may be focally present or the predominant feature. Smears of epithelioid leiomyosarcomas may be confused with carcinomas. Cell block preparations (Figure 7–70) are usually helpful. In difficult cases, or ones with no known history, immunoperoxidase stains demonstrating vimentin (Figure 7–71) and desmin (Figure 7–72) are supportive of myogenic differentiation.

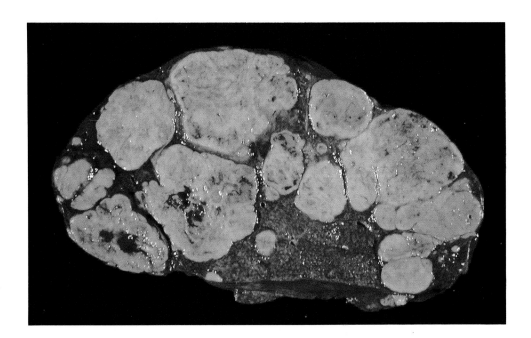

FIGURE 7–66 Metastatic leiomyosarcoma. Tumor nodules are large and bulky with rounded pushing borders.

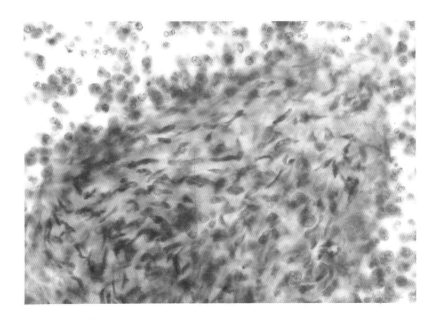

FIGURE 7–67 Metastatic leiomyosarcoma. Tumor occurs in large fragments of cellular spindle cells with obscured nuclear detail. (Papanicolaou, ×160.)

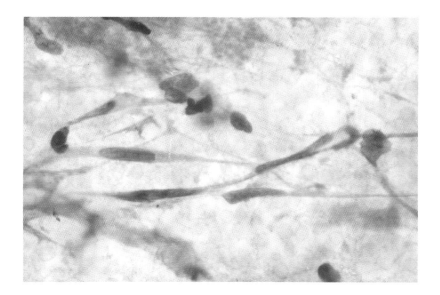

FIGURE 7–68 Metastatic leiomyosarcoma. Detached single cells better illustrate the oval cigar-shaped nuclei with rounded ends and bipolar cytoplasm. (Papanicolaou, ×160.)

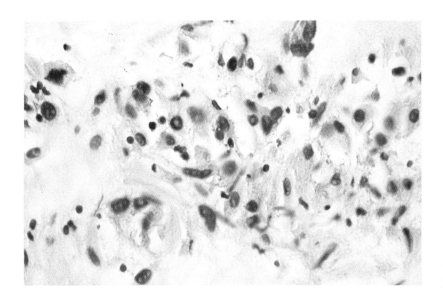

FIGURE 7–69 Metastatic leiomyosarcoma. Cell block preparation demonstrating epithelioid characteristics manifested by round polygonal cells with round to oval nuclei and pink cytoplasm. (Hematoxylin & eosin, ×160.)

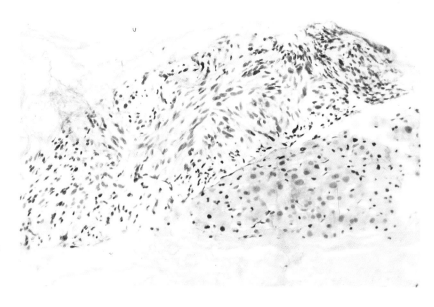

FIGURE 7–70 Metastatic leiomyosarcoma. Cell block preparation showing large fragment of interweaving fascicles of spindle cells adjacent to reactive hepatocytes. (Hematoxylin & eosin, ×64.)

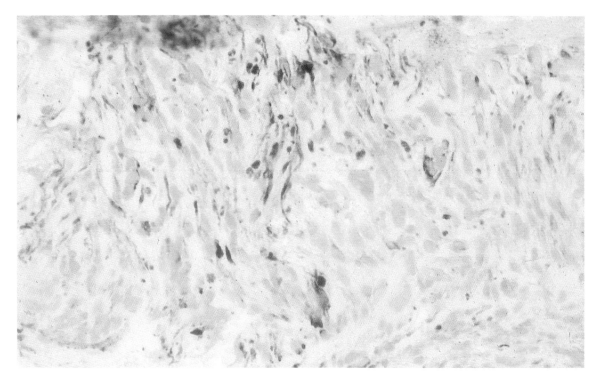

FIGURE 7–71 Metastatic leiomyosarcoma. The tumor is focally positive for vimentin. (Immunoperoxidase, ×100.)

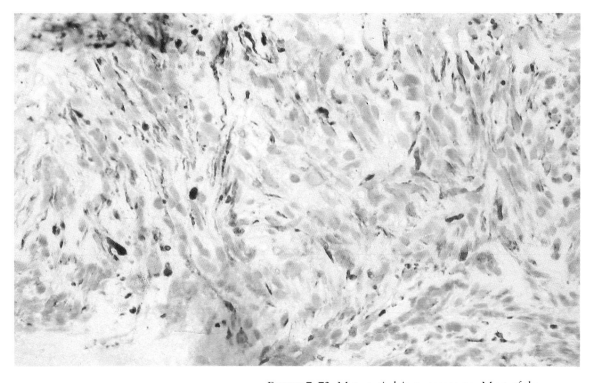

FIGURE 7–72 Metastatic leiomyosarcoma. Most of the tumor cells are positive for desmin, which supports myogenic differentiation. (Immunoperoxidase, ×100.)

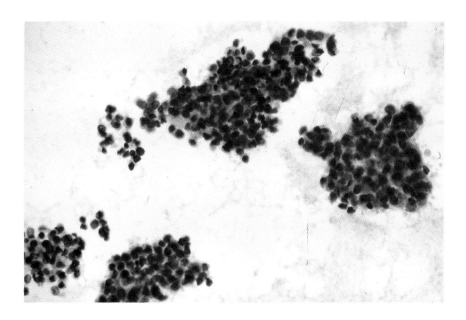

FIGURE 7–73 Metastatic granulosa cell tumor. Tumor cells occur in irregular cohesive nests and have a monotonous uniform appearance similar to neuroendocrine tumors. (Papanicolaou, ×100.)

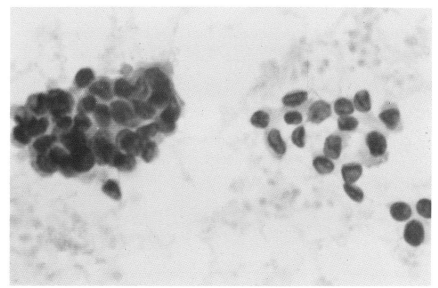

FIGURE 7–74 Metastatic granulosa cell tumor. The more dishesive group of cells demonstrates characteristic nuclear grooving. (Papanicolaou, ×160.)

RARE

Granulosa Cell Tumor

Granulosa cell tumor is a low-grade malignancy that tends to recur locally and remain within the pelvis and abdomen.[13] Distant metastases are vary rare but have been reported in the lungs, liver, bone, and brain, sometimes many years after the initial diagnosis.[13]

Aspirate smears show cellular, cohesive clusters composed of small hyperchromatic, rather uniform cells (Figure 7–73) that on low to medium power magnification resemble a neuroendocrine tumor, especially carcinoid tumor. Higher power magnification (Figure 7–74), however, reveals a dense, coarse chromatin without the typical neuroendocrine "salt and pepper" chromatin distribution of carcinoid tumors, and nuclear grooves characteristic of granulosa cell tumor are usually apparent.

Female Adnexal Tumor of Probable Wolffian Origin

Female adnexal tumor of probable Wolffian origin (FATPWO) is a rare tumor of the adnexa that occurs in women of all ages.[14] It is most often a benign lesion discovered incidentally, but there have been reports of malignant behavior.[15,16] Histologically (Figure 7–75), the tumor is classically composed of a sievelike tubulocystic array of glands lined by cuboidal to columnar cells. In the case of metastatic FATPWO to the liver we diagnosed, the aspirate smears showed degenerated clusters of glandular cells not typical of bile duct epithelium in a background of abundant necrosis (Figure 7–76). With the patient's history, these groups were suspicious but not diagnostic of metastatic disease. The cell block (Figure 7–77), on the other hand, showed a large fragment of tissue composed of bland-appearing glands lined by columnar cells consistent with metastatic FATPWO.

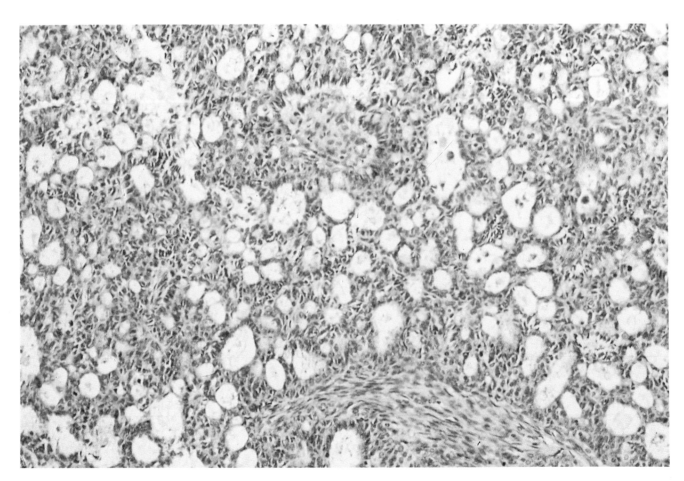

FIGURE 7–75 Metastatic female adnexal tumor of probable Wolffian origin. A histologic section demonstrates the characteristic sievelike glandular pattern. (Hematoxylin & eosin, ×40).

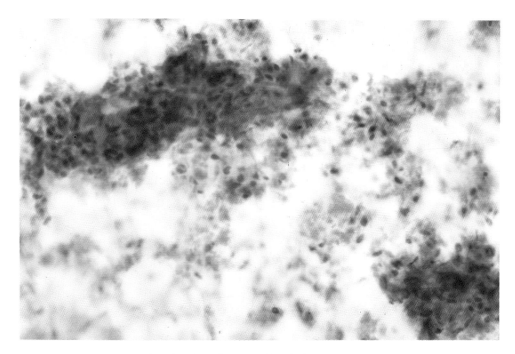

FIGURE 7–76 Metastatic female adnexal tumor of probable
Wolffian origin. Cluster of degenerated epithelial cells in a
background of necrosis. (Papanicolaou, ×100.)

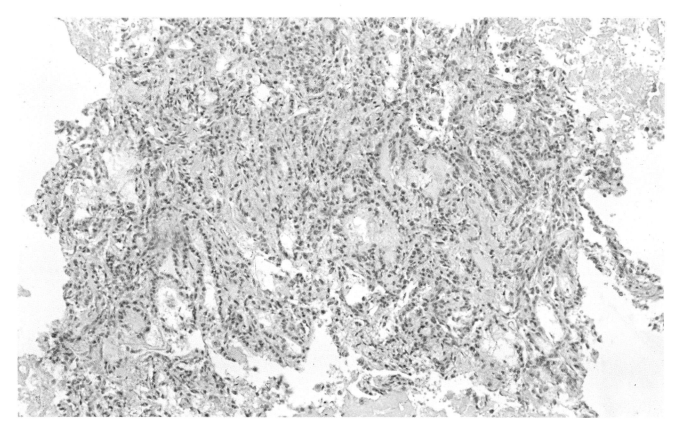

FIGURE 7–77 Metastatic female adnexal tumor of probable
Wolffian origin (FATPWO). A cell block preparation beautifully demonstrates viable metastatic tumor consistent with a
metastatic FATPWO. (Hematoxylin & eosin, ×40.)

REFERENCES

1. Edmondson HA, Craig JR. Neoplasms of the liver. In: Schiff L, Schiff ER, eds. Diseases of the liver. 6th ed. Philadelphia: JB Lippincott, 1987;1116–1118.

2. DeMent SH, Mann RB, Staal SP, et al. Primary lymphomas of the liver: report of six cases and review of the literature. Am J Clin Pathol 1987;88:255–263.

3. Kanel GC, Konila J. Atlas of liver pathology. Philadelphia: WB Saunders, 1992;213–215.

4. Soderstrom N. Fine-needle aspiration biopsy. Stockholm: Almqvist and Wiksell, 1966.

5. Orell SR, Sterrett GF, Walters MN-I, Whitaker D. Manual and atlas of fine needle aspiration cytology. Edinburgh: Churchill Livingstone, 1986;46.

6. Koss GL, Woyke S, Olszewski W. The skin and soft tissue. In: Aspiration biopsy. Cytologic interpretation and histologic bases. New York: Igaku-Shoin, 1984; 250–284.

7. Tao L-C. Transabdominal fine-needle aspiration biopsy. New York: Agaku-Shoin, 1990;80.

8. Hajdu SI, Hajdee EO. Malignant melanoma. In: Cytopathology of sarcomas and other nonepithelial malignant tumors. Philadelphia: WB Saunders, 1976; 305–322.

9. Wick MR, ed. Pathology of unusual malignant cutaneous tumors. In: Clinical and biochemical analysis. Vol. 20. 1985;293.

10. Gown AM, Vogel AM, Hoak D, McNut MA. Monoclonal antibodies specific for melanocytic tumors distinguish subpopulations of melanocytes. Am J Pathol 1986;123:195–203.

11. Pitman MB, Szyfelbein WM. The significance of endothelium in the FNA diagnosis of hepatocellular carcinoma. Diagn Cytopathol (in press).

12. Craig JR, Peters RL, Edmondson HA. Tumors of the liver and intrahepatic bile ducts. Washington, DC: Armed Forces Institute of Pathology, 1987;234.

13. Scully RE. Tumors of the ovary and maldeveloped gonads. Fascicle 16, 2nd series. Washington, DC: AFIP, 1979;169.

14. Kariminejad MH, Scully RE. Female adnexal tumor of probable Wolffian origin. A distinctive pathologic entity. Cancer 1973;31:671–677.

15. Taxy JB, Battifore H. Female adnexal tumor of probable Wolffian origin. Evidence for a low grade malignancy. Cancer 1976;37:2349–2354.

16. Abbot RL, Barlogie B, Schmidt WA. Metastasizing malignant jaxatovarian tumor with terminal hypercalcemia: a case report. Cancer 1981;48:860–865.

Index